Study Guide to Accompany

The Human Body in Health & Disease

Fifth Edition

Linda Swisher, RN, EdD

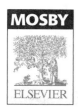

MOSBY

ELSEVIER

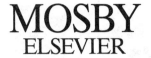

11830 Westline Industrial Drive
St. Louis, Missouri 63146

Study Guide to accompany The Human
Body in Health & Disease, Fifth Edition

ISBN: 978-0-323-05487-4

Notice

Neither the Publisher nor the Authors assume any responsibility for any loss or injury and/or
damage to persons or property arising out of or related to any use of the material contained in
this book. It is the responsibility of the treating practitioner, relying on independent expertise
and knowledge of the patient, to determine the best treatment and method of application for
the patient.

The Publisher

ISBN: 978-0-323-05487-4

Acquisitions Editor: Jeff Downing
Developmental Editor: Karen C. Turner
Editorial Assistant: Jennifer Shropshire
Publishing Services Manager: Deborah L. Vogel
Senior Project Manager: Ann Rogers
Design Manager: Mark Oberkrom

Printed in the United States of America
Last digit is the print number: 9 8 7 6 5 4 3 2

Acknowledgments

I wish to express my appreciation to the staff of Mosby, Inc., especially Tom Wilhelm, Jeff Downing, Karen Turner, and Jennifer Shropshire for opening the door and assisting me with this text. My continued admiration and gratitude to Kevin Patton and Gary Thibodeau for an outstanding text. Your time and dedication to science education will, I hope, inspire potential caregivers and improve the quality of health care for the future.

To my family and Brian, my thanks for your assistance and support.

To Bill, who is always there, my thanks for the whispers of inspiration.

Finally, to the designer of the human body, this book is dedicated. What a miraculous creation!

Linda Swisher, RN, EdD

Preface

TO THE INSTRUCTOR

This Study Guide is designed to help your students master basic anatomy and physiology. It works in two ways.

First, the section of the preface titled "To the Student," contains detailed instructions on:

- How to achieve good grades in anatomy and physiology
- How to read the textbook
- How to use the exercises in this Study Guide
- How to use visual memory as a learning tool
- How to use mnemonic devices as learning aids
- How to prepare for an examination
- How to take an examination
- How to find out why questions were missed on an examination

Second, the Study Guide itself contains features that facilitate learning:

1. LEARNING OBJECTIVES, designed to break down the process of learning into small units. The questions in this Study Guide have been developed to help the student master the learning objectives identified at the beginning of each chapter in the text. The Guide is also sequenced to correspond to key areas of each chapter. A variety of questions have been prepared to cover the material effectively and expose the student to multiple learning approaches.

2. CROSSWORD PUZZLES, to encourage the use of new vocabulary words and emphasize the proper spelling of these terms.

3. OPTIONAL APPLICATION QUESTIONS, particularly targeted for the health occupations student, but appropriate for any student of anatomy and physiology because questions are based entirely on information contained within the chapter.

4. DIAGRAMS with key features marked by numbers for identification. Students can easily check their work by comparing the diagram in the workbook with the equivalent figure in the text.

5. PAGE NUMBER REFERENCES in the answer sections. Each answer is cross-referenced to the appropriate text page. In addition, questions are grouped into specific topics that correspond to the text. Each major topic of the Study Guide provides references to specific areas of the text, so that students having difficulty with a particular grouping of questions have a specific reference area to assist them with remedial work. This is of great assistance to both instructor and student, because remedial work is made easier and more effective when the area of weakness is identified accurately.

These features should make mastery of the material a rewarding experience for both instructor and student.

TO THE STUDENT

How to Achieve Good Grades in Anatomy and Physiology

This Study Guide is designed to help you be successful in learning anatomy and physiology. Before you begin using the Study Guide, read the following suggestions. Successful students understand effective study techniques and have good study habits.

How to Read the Textbook

Keep up with the reading assignments. Read the textbook assignment before the instructor covers the material in a lecture. If you have failed to read the assignment beforehand, you may not grasp what the instructor is talking about in the lecture. When you read, do the following:

1. As you finish reading a sentence, ask yourself if you understand it. If you do not, put a question mark in the margin by that sentence. If the instructor does not clarify the material in lecture, ask him or her to explain it to you further.

2. Do the learning objectives in the text. A learning objective is a specific task that you are expected to be able to do after you have read a chapter. It sets specific goals for the student and breaks down learning into small units. It emphasizes the key points that the author is making in the chapter.

3. Underline and make notes in the margin to highlight key ideas, mark something you need to reinforce at a later time, or indicate things that you do not understand.

4. If you come to a word you do not understand, look it up in a dictionary. Write the word on one side of an index card and its definition on the other side. Carry these cards with you, and when you have a spare minute, use them like flash cards. If you do not know how to spell or pronounce a word, you will have a hard time remembering it.

5. Carefully study each diagram and illustration as you read. Many students ignore these aids. The author included them to help students understand the material.

6. Summarize what you read. After finishing a paragraph, try to restate the main ideas. Do this again when you finish the chapter. Identify and mentally restate the main concepts of the chapter. Check to see if you are correct. In short, be an active reader. Do not just stare at a page or read it superficially.

7. Finally, attack each unit of learning with a positive mental attitude. Motivation and perseverance are prime factors in achieving good grades. The combination of your instructor, the text, the Study Guide, and your dedicated work will lead to success in anatomy and physiology.

How to Use the Exercises in this Study Guide

After you have read a chapter and learned all of the new words, begin working with the Study Guide. Read the overview of the chapter, which summarizes the main points.

Familiarize yourself with the "Topics for Review" section, which emphasizes the learning objectives outlined in the text. Complete the questions and diagrams in the Study Guide. After completing the exercises in a chapter, you can check your answers in the back of the book. Each answer is referenced to the appropriate text page. Additionally, questions are grouped into specific topics that correspond to the text. Each major topic of the Study and Review Guide provides references to specific areas of the text, so if you are having difficulty with a particular grouping of questions you have a specific reference area to assist you with remedial work. This feature allows you to identify your area of weakness accurately. A variety of questions are offered throughout the Study Guide to help you cover the material effectively. The following examples are among the exercises that have been included to assist you.

Multiple Choice Questions

Multiple choice questions will have only one correct answer for you to select from the several possibilities presented. There are two types of multiple choice questions that you need to be acquainted with:

1. "None of the above is correct" questions. These questions test your ability to recall rather than recognize the correct answer. You would select the "none of the above" choice only if all the other choices in that particular question were incorrect.

2. Sequence questions. These questions test your ability to arrange a list of structures in the correct order. In this type of question, you are asked to determine the sequence of the structures given in the various choices, and then you are to select the structure listed that would be third in that sequence, as in this example.

    Which one of the following structures is the third through which food passes?

A. Stomach
B. Mouth
C. Large intestine
D. Esophagus
E. Anus

The correct answer is *A.*

Matching Questions

Matching questions ask the student to select the correct answer from a list of terms and to write that answer in the space provided.

True or False Questions

True or false questions ask you to write "T" in the answer space if you agree with that statement. If you disagree with the statement, you will circle the incorrect word(s) and write the correct word(s) in the answer space.

Identify the Term that Does Not Belong

In questions that ask you to identify the incorrect term, three words are given that relate to each other in structure or function, and one more word is included that has no relationship, or has an opposing relationship to the other three terms. You are asked to circle the term that does not relate to the others. An example might be: iris, cornea, stapes, retina. You would circle the word *stapes* because all other terms refer to the eye.

Fill-in-the-Blank Questions

Fill-in-the-blank questions ask you to recall one or moremissing word and insert them into the answer blanks. These questions may involve sentences or paragraphs.

Application Questions

Application questions ask you to make judgments about a situation based on the information in the chapter. These questions may concern how you would respond to a situation or ask you to suggest a possible diagnosis for a set of symptoms.

Charts

Several charts have been included that correspond to figures in the text. Areas have been omitted so that you can fill them in and test your recall of these important concepts.

Word Find Puzzles

The Study Guide includes word find puzzles that allow you to identify key terms in the chapter in an interesting and challenging way.

Crossword Puzzles

Vocabulary words from the "New Words" section at the end of each chapter of the text have been developed into crossword puzzles. This encourages recall and proper spelling. Occasionally, an exercise uses scrambled words to encourage recall and spelling.

Labeling Exercises

Labeling exercises present diagrams with parts that are not identified. For each of these diagrams, you are to print the name of each numbered part on the appropriately numbered line. You may choose to further distinguish the structures by coloring them with a variety of colors. After you have written down the names of the structures to be identified, check your answers. When it comes time to review for an examination, you can place a sheet of paper over your answers to test yourself.

After completing the exercises in the Study Guide, check your answers. If they are not correct, refer to the answers page and review it for further clarification. If you still do not understand the question or the answer, ask your instructor for further explanation or assistance.

If you have difficulty with several questions from one section, refer to the pages listed at the end of the section. After reviewing the section, try to answer the questions again. If you are still having difficulty, talk to your instructor.

Check Your Knowledge

This section selects questions from throughout the chapter to provide you with a final review. This mini-test gives you an overview of your knowledge of the entire chapter after completing all of the other sections. It emphasizes the main concepts of the unit, but should not be attempted until the specific topics of the chapter have been mastered.

How to Use Visual Memory

Visual memory is another important tool in learning. If I asked you to picture an elephant in your mind, with all its external parts labeled, you could do that easily. Visual memory is a powerful key to learning. Whenever possible, try to build a memory picture. Remember: a picture is worth a thousand words.

Visual memory works especially well with the sequencing of items, such as circulatory pathways and the passage of air or food. Students who try to learn sequencing by memorizing a list of words do poorly on examinations. If they forget one word in the sequence, they then may forget the remaining words as well. With a memory picture you can pick out the important features.

How to Use Mnemonic Devices

Mnemonic devices are little jingles that you memorize to help you remember things. If you make up your own, they will stick with you longer. Here are three examples of such devices:

"On Old Olympus' towering tops a Finn and German viewed some hops." This one is used to remember the cranial nerves. Each word begins with the same letter as does the name of one of the nerves: . olfactory, optic, oculomotor, trochlear, trigeminal, abducens, facial, auditory, glossopharyngeal, vagus, sensory (accessory), and hypoglossal.

"C. Hopkins CaFe where they serve Mg NaCl." This mnemonic device reminds you of the chemical symbols for the biologically important electrolytes: carbon, hydrogen, oxygen, phosphorus, potassium, iodine, nitrogen, sulfur, calcium, iron, magnesium, sodium, chlorine. "Roy G. Biv." This mnemonic device helps you remember the colors of the visible light spectrum: red, orange, yellow, green, blue, indigo, violet.

How to Prepare for an Examination

Prepare far in advance for an examination. Actually, your preparation for an examination should begin on the first day of class. Keeping up with your assignments daily makes the final preparation for an examination much easier. You should begin your final preparation at least three nights before the test. Last-minute studying usually means poor results and limited retention.

1. Make sure that you understand and can answer all of the learning objectives for the chapter on which you are being tested.

2. Review the appropriate questions in this Study Guide. Review is something that you should do after every class and at the end of every study session. It is important to keep going over the material until you have a thorough understanding of the chapter and rapid recall of its contents. If review becomes a daily habit, studying for the actual examination will not be difficult. Go through each question and

write down an answer. Do the same with the labeling of each structure on the appropriate diagrams. If you have already done this as part of your daily review, cover the answers with a piece of paper and quiz yourself again.

3. Check the answers that you have written down against the correct answers in the back of the Study Guide. Go back and study the areas in the text that refer to questions that you missed and then try to answer those questions again. If you still cannot answer a question or label a structure correctly, ask your instructor for help.

4. As you read a chapter, ask yourself what questions you would ask if you were writing a test on that unit. You will most likely ask yourself many of the questions that will show up on your examinations.

5. Get a good night's sleep before the test. Staying up late and upsetting your biorhythms will only make you less efficient during the test.

How to Take an Examination

The Day of the Test

1. Get up early enough to avoid rushing. Eat appropriately. Your body needs fuel, but a heavy meal just before a test is not a good idea.

2. Keep calm. Briefly look over your notes. If you have prepared for the test properly, there will be no need for last-minute cramming.

3. Make certain that you have everything you need for the test: pens, pencils, test sheets, and so forth.

4. Allow enough time to get to the examination site. Missing your bus, getting stuck in traffic, or being unable to find a parking space will not put you in a good frame of mind to do well on the examination.

During the Examination

1. Pay careful attention to the instructions for the test.

2. Note any corrections.

3. Budget your time so that you will be able to finish the test.

4. Ask the instructor for clarification if you do not understand a question or an instruction.

5. Concentrate on your own test paper and do not allow yourself to be distracted by others in the room.

Hints for Taking a Multiple-Choice Test

1. Read each question carefully. Pay attention to each word.

2. Cross out obviously wrong choices and think about those that are left.

3. Go through the test once, quickly answering the questions you are sure of; then go back over the test and answer the rest of the questions.

4. Fill in the answer spaces completely and make your marks heavy. Erase answers completely if you make a mistake.

5. If you must guess, stick with your first hunch. Most often, students will change right answers to wrong ones.

6. If you will not be penalized for guessing, do not leave any blanks.

Hints for Taking an Essay Test

1. Budget time for each question.

2. Write legibly and try to spell words correctly.

3. Be concise, complete, and specific. Do not be repetitious or long-winded.

4.   Organize your answer in an outline—this helps not only you but also the person who grades the test.

5.   Answer each question as thoroughly as you can, but leave some room for possible additions.

Hints for Taking a Laboratory Practical Examination

Students often have a hard time with this kind of test. Visual memory is very important here. To put it simply, you must be able to identify every structure you have studied. If you are unable to identify a structure, then you will be unable to answer any questions about that structure.

Possible questions that could appear on an examination of this type might include:

1.   Identification of a structure, organ, or feature.

2.   Identification of the function of a structure, organ, or feature.

3.   Sequence questions for air flow, passage of food or urine, and so forth.

4.   Disease questions (for example, if an organ fails, what disease will result?).

How to Find Out Why Questions Were Missed on an Examination

After the Examination

Go over your test after it has been scored to see what you missed and why you missed it. You can pick up important clues that will help you on future examinations. Ask yourself these questions:

1.   Did I miss questions because I did not read them carefully?

2.   Did I miss questions because I had gaps in my knowledge?

3.   Did I miss questions because I could not determine scientific words?

4.   Did I miss questions because I did not have good visual memory of things?

Be sure to go back and learn the things you did not know. Chances are these topics will come up on the final examination.

Your grades in other classes will improve as well when you apply these study methods. Learning should be fun. With these helpful hints and this Study Guide you should be able to achieve the grades you desire. Good luck!

Contents

CHAPTER 1

An Introduction to the Structure and Function of the Body

A command of terminology is necessary for a student to be successful in any area of science. This chapter defines the terminology and concepts that are basic to the field of anatomy and physiology. Building a firm foundation in these language skills will assist you with all future chapters.

The study of anatomy and physiology involves the structure and function of an organism and the relationship of its parts. It begins with a basic organization of the body into different structural levels. Beginning with the smallest level (the cell) and progressing to the largest, most complex level (the system), this chapter familiarizes you with the terminology and the levels of organization needed to facilitate the study of the body as a part or as a whole.

It is also important to be able to identify and describe specific body areas or regions as we progress in our study of this field. The anatomical position is used as a reference position when dissecting the body into planes, regions, or cavities. The terminology defined in this chapter allows you to describe the areas efficiently and accurately.

Finally, the process of homeostasis is reviewed. This state of relative constancy in the chemical composition of body fluids is necessary for good health. In fact, the very survival of the body depends on the successful maintenance of homeostasis.

TOPICS FOR REVIEW

Before progressing to Chapter 2, you should have an understanding of the structural levels of organization; the planes, regions, and cavities of the body; the terminology used to describe these areas; and the concept of homeostasis as it relates to the survival of the species.

STRUCTURAL LEVELS OF ORGANIZATION

Match each term on the left with its corresponding description on the right.

____D____ 1. Organism   A. Many similar cells that act together to perform a common function

____e____ 2. Cells   B. The most complex units that make up the body

____a____ 3. Tissue   C. A group of several different kinds of tissues arranged to perform a special function

____c____ 4. Organ   D. Denotes a living thing

____b____ 5. Systems   E. The smallest "living" units of structure and function in the body

▶ *If you had difficulty with this section, review pages 3-6.*

ANATOMICAL POSITION

Match each term on the left with its corresponding description on the right.

B C 6. Body   A. At the sides

a 7. Arms   B. Face upward

e 8. Feet   C. Erect

D 9. Prone   D. Face downward

a 10. Supine   E. Forward

 If you had difficulty with this section, review pages 6-7.

ANATOMICAL DIRECTIONS

Planes or Body Sections

Fill in the crossword puzzle.

ACROSS
12. Lower or below
13. Horizontal plane
16. Toward the midline of the body

DOWN
11. Upper or above
14. Front (abdominal side)
15. Toward the side of the body
17. Farthest from the point of origin of a body point

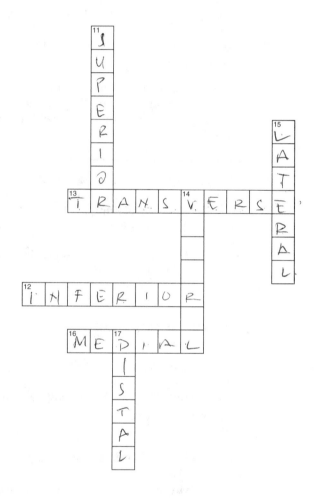

Circle the correct answer.

18. The stomach is (*superior* or *inferior*) to the diaphragm.

19. The nose is located on the (*anterior* or *posterior*) surface of the body.

20. The lungs lie (*medial* or *lateral*) to the heart.

21. The elbow lies (*proximal* or *distal*) to the forearm.

22. The skin is (*superficial* or *deep*) to the muscles below it.

23. A midsagittal plane divides the body into (*equal* or *unequal*) parts.

24. A frontal plane divides the body into (*anterior and posterior* or *superior and inferior*) sections.

25. A transverse plane divides the body into (*right and left* or *upper and lower*) sections.

26. A coronal plane may also be referred to as a (*sagittal* or *frontal*) plane.

▶ *If you had difficulty with this section, review pages 7-8.*

BODY CAVITIES

Match each term with its body cavity location and write A or B in the answer blank.

A. Ventral cavity   B. Dorsal cavity

___A___ 27. Thoracic

___B___ 28. Cranial

___A___ 29. Abdominal

___A___ 30. Pelvic

___A___ 31. Mediastinum

___B___ 32. Spinal

___A___ 33. Pleural

▶ *If you had difficulty with this section, review page 10.*

BODY REGIONS

Circle the word in each word group that does not belong.

34. Axial   Head   Trunk   Extremities

35. Axillary   Cephalic   Brachial   Antecubital

36. Frontal   Orbital   Plantar   Nasal

37. (Carpal)   Crural   Plantar   Pedal }   part of foot

38. Cranial   Occipital   Tarsal   Temporal

▶ *If you had difficulty with this section, review pages 11-13.*

For each of the following statements, write "T" in the answer blank if the statement is true. If the statement is false, circle the incorrect word(s) and write the correct word(s) in the answer blank.

_____ 39. The term *autopsy* comes from the Greek words auto (self) and opsis (view).

_____ 40. Autopsies are usually performed in four stages.

_____ 41. In the first stage of an autopsy, the exterior of the body is examined for abnormalities such as wounds or scars.

_____ 42. The face, arms, and legs are usually dissected during the second stage of an autopsy.

_____ 43. Microscopic examination of tissues occurs during all stages of an autopsy.

_____ 44. Tests to analyze the chemical content of body fluids or to determine the presence of infectious organisms may also be performed during an autopsy.

▷ _If you had difficulty with this section, review page 11._

THE BALANCE OF BODY FUNCTIONS

Fill in the blanks.

45. _____ depends on the body's ability to maintain or restore homeostasis.

46. _Homeostasis_ is the term used to describe the relative constancy of the body's ___internal_____ ___environment_____.

47. During exercise, homeostasis is disrupted and may cause the body's temperature to ___sweat___ ___rise___.

48. Changes and functions that occur during the early years are called ___developmental_____.

49. Changes and functions that occur after young adulthood are called ___aging_____.

50. Homeostatic control mechanisms are categorized as either ___negative_____ or ___positive_____ feedback loops.

51. Negative feedback loops are ___stimulizing stabilizes___ mechanisms.

52. Positive feedback control loops are ___stimulizing_____.

▷ _If you had difficulty with this section, review pages 13-17._

APPLYING WHAT YOU KNOW

53. Mrs. Hunt has had an appendectomy. The nurse is preparing to change the dressing. She knows that the appendix is located in the right iliac inguinal region, the distal portion extending at an angle into the hypogastric region. Place an X on the diagram where the nurse will place the dressing.

54. Mrs. Wiedeke noticed a lump in her breast. Dr. Reeder noted on her chart that a small mass was located in the left breast medial to the nipple. Place an X where Mrs. Wiedeke's lump would be located.

55. Heather was injured in a bicycle accident. X-ray films revealed that she had a fracture of the right patella. A cast was applied beginning at the distal femoral region and extending to the pedal region. Place one X where Heather's cast begins and another where it ends.

56.　Word Find

Find and circle 18 terms presented in this chapter. Words may be spelled top to bottom, bottom to top, right to left, left to right, or diagonally.

Anatomy
Atrophy
Homeostasis
Medial
Mediastinum
Organ
Organization
Physiology
Pleural

Posterior
Proximal
Sagittal
Superficial
Superior
System
Thoracic
Tissue
Ventral

```
N H L T E B W N G N M M Y X A
O O H A V U U C L W E P N G L
I M U N I T S A I D E M W A L
T E R T V C T S I C J S R T K
A O N O P T I A I W A T Y R H
Z S Q S I R L F A T N R G O W
I T W G P R O I R E T S O P F
N A A Z J E E X V E E H L H Z
A S N L M C T P I C P D O Y T
G I C A Y U O X U M N U I V P
R S M R T N U K B S A Y S V M
O R C U R O I R B S Q L Y U G
L H X E M P M E T S Y S H V S
U W L L Q D U Y Y N E E P J B
Q N Z P K D B O D C G I N J A
```

DID YOU KNOW?

Many animals produce tears but only humans weep as a result of emotional stress.

CHECK YOUR KNOWLEDGE

Multiple Choice

Circle the correct answer.

1. The body's ability to respond continuously to changes in the environment and maintain consistency in the internal environment is called:
   A. Homeostasis
   B. Superficial
   C. Structural levels
   D. None of the above

2. The regions frequently used by health professionals to locate pain or tumors divides the abdomen into four basic areas called:
   A. Planes
   B. Cavities
   C. Pleural
   D. Quadrants

3. Which of the following organs or structures does *not* lie within the mediastinum?
   A. Thymus
   B. Liver
   C. Esophagus
   D. Trachea

4. A lengthwise plane running from front to back that divides the body into right and left sides is called:
   A. Transverse
   B. Coronal
   C. Frontal
   D. Sagittal

5. A study of the functions of living organisms and their parts is called:
   A. Physiology
   B. Chemistry
   C. Biology
   D. None of the above

6. The thoracic portion of the ventral body cavity is separated from the abdominopelvic portion by a muscle called the:
    A. Latissimus dorsi
    B. Rectus femoris
    C. Diaphragm
    D. Pectoralis

7. An organization of varying numbers and kinds of organs arranged together to perform a complex function is called a:
    A. Cell
    B. Tissue
    C. System
    D. Region

8. The plane that divides superior from inferior is known as the _____ plane.
    A. Transverse
    B. Sagittal
    C. Frontal
    D. None of the above

9. Which of the following structures does *not* lie within the abdominal cavity?
    A. Spleen
    B. Most of the small intestine
    C. Urinary bladder
    D. Stomach

10. Which of the following is an example of an upper abdominal region?
    A. Right iliac region
    B. Left hypochondriac region
    C. Left lumbar region
    D. Hypogastric region

11. The dorsal body cavity contains components of the:
    A. Reproductive system
    B. Digestive system
    C. Respiratory system
    D. Nervous system

12. Which of the following organs is *not* found in the pelvic cavity?
    A. Bladder
    B. Stomach
    C. Rectum
    D. Colon

13. Similar cells acting together to perform a common function exist at a level of organization called a/an:
    A. Organ
    B. Chemical
    C. Tissue
    D. System

14. Which of the following planes would be considered coronal?
    A. A plane that divides the body into anterior and posterior portions
    B. A plane that divides the body into upper and lower portions
    C. A plane that divides the body into right and left sides
    D. A plane that divides the body into superficial and deep portions

15. If your reference point is "nearest to the trunk of the body" versus "farthest from the trunk of the body," where does the elbow lie in relation to the wrist?
    A. Anterior
    B. Posterior
    C. Distal
    D. Proximal

16. In the anatomical position:
    A. The dorsal body cavity is anterior to the ventral
    B. Palms face toward the back of the body
    C. The body is erect
    D. All of the above

17. The buttocks are often used as intramuscular injection sites. This region can be called:
    A. Sacral
    B. Buccal
    C. Cutaneous
    D. Gluteal

18. In the human body, the chest region:
    A. Can be referred to as the thoracic cavity
    B. Is a component of the ventral body cavity
    C. Contains the mediastinum
    D. All of the above

19. Which of the following is *not* a component of the axial subdivision of the body?
    A. Upper extremity
    B. Neck
    C. Trunk
    D. Head

20. The scientific study of disease is:
    A. Dissection
    B. Volar
    C. Pathology
    D. Pathogens

Matching

Match each term in column A with the most appropriate term in column B. Write the corresponding letter in the answer blank. (Only one answer is correct for each.)

Column A

_____ 21. Ventral
__B__ 22. Skin
__J__ 23. Transverse
_____ 24. Anatomy
__H__ 25. Superficial
__C__ 26. Pleural
__D__ 27. Appendicular
__I__ 28. Posterior
__A__ 29. Midsagittal
__G__ 30. System

Column B

A. Equal
B. Cutaneous
C. Lung
D. Extremities
E. Respiratory
F. Anterior
G. Structure
H. Surface
I. Back
J. Horizontal

Fill in the Blanks

Complete these statements.

31. A systemic approach to discovery is known as the _____.

32. A tentative explanation in research is known as a _____.

33. The testing of a hypothesis is_____.

34. In clinical trials, a group getting a drug is the _____.

35. In clinical trials, a group getting a substitute is the _____.

DORSAL AND VENTRAL BODY CAVITIES

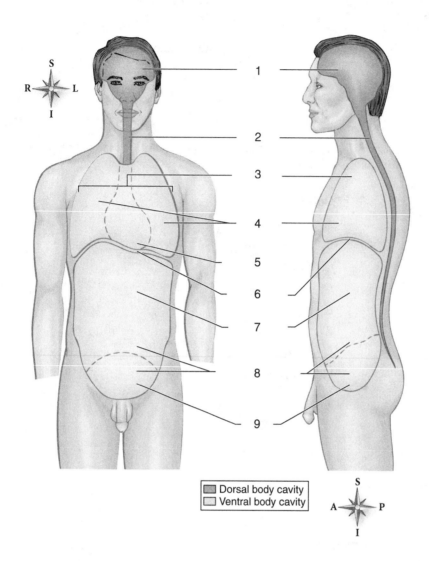

Dorsal body cavity
Ventral body cavity

1. _____cranial_____
2. _____spine_____
3. _____thoracic_____
4. _____pleural_____
5. _____mediastenum_____
6. _____diaphragm_____
7. _____abdominal_____
8. _____abdominopelvic_____
9. _____pelvic_____

DIRECTIONS AND PLANES OF THE BODY

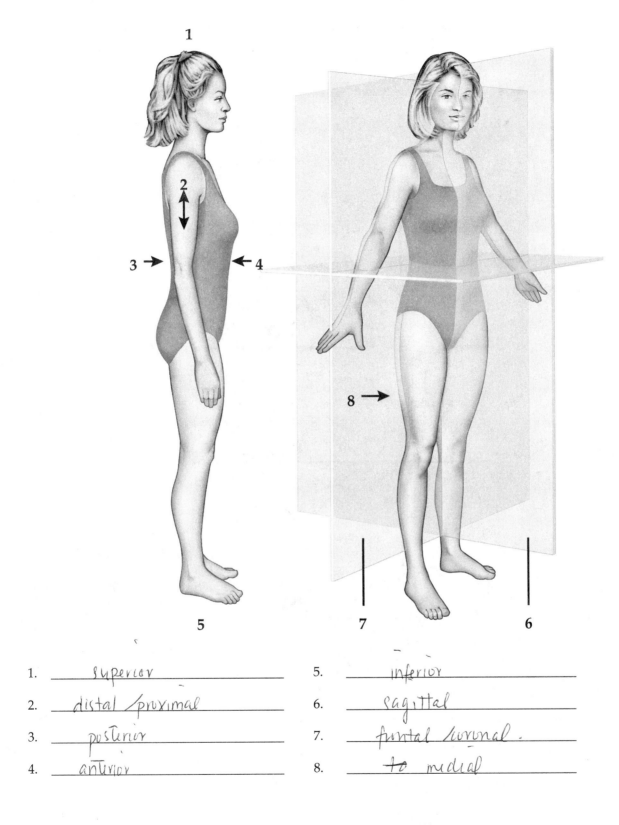

1. _____Superior_____
2. _____distal /proximal_____
3. _____posterior_____
4. _____anterior_____
5. _____inferior_____
6. _____sagittal_____
7. _____frontal coronal._____
8. _____to medial_____

REGIONS OF THE ABDOMEN

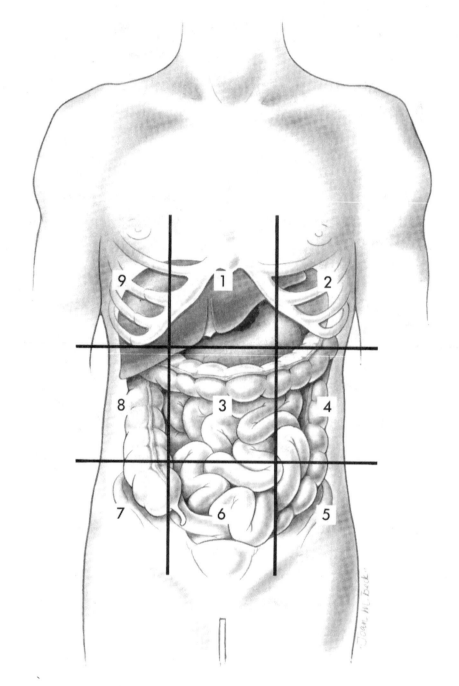

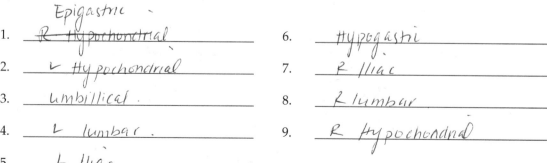

Epigastric

1. ~~R~~ Hypochondrial

2. L Hypochondrial

3. umbillical.

4. L lumbar.

5. L Iliac

6. Hypogastri

7. R Iliac

8. L lumbar

9. R Hypochondral

CHAPTER 2

Chemistry of Life

Although anatomy can be studied without knowledge of the principles of chemistry, it is hard to imagine having an understanding of physiology without a basic comprehension of chemical reactions in the body. Trillions of cells make up the various levels of organization in the body. Our health and survival depends upon the proper chemical maintenance in the cytoplasm of our cells.

Chemists use the terms *elements* or *compounds* to describe all of the substances (matter) in and around us. What distinguishes these two terms is their basic structure. An element cannot be broken down. A compound, on the other hand, is made up of two or more elements and can be broken down into the elements that form it.

Organic and inorganic compounds are equally important to our survival. Without organic compounds, such as carbohydrates, proteins, and fats, and inorganic compounds, such as water, we could not sustain life.

Because we cannot see many of the chemical reactions that take place daily in our bodies, it is sometimes difficult to comprehend the principles involved in initiating them. Chemicals are responsible for directing virtually all of our bodily functions. Therefore, it is important to master the fundamental concepts of chemistry in order to understand physiology.

TOPICS FOR REVIEW

Before progressing to Chapter 3, you should have an understanding of the basic chemical reactions in the body and the fundamental concepts of biochemistry.

LEVELS OF CHEMICAL ORGANIZATION

Multiple Choice

Circle the correct answer.

1. Which of the following is *not* a subatomic particle?
   A. Proton
   B. Electron
   C. Isotope
   D. Neutron

2. Electrons move about within certain limits called:
   A. Energy levels
   B. Orbitals
   C. Chemical bonding
   D. Shells

3. The number of protons in the nucleus is an atom's:
   A. Atomic mass
   B. Atomic energy level
   C. Atomic number
   D. None of the above

4. The number of protons and neutrons combined is the atom's:
   A. Atomic mass
   B. Atomic energy level
   C. Orbit
   D. Chemical bonding

5. Which of the following is *not* one of the major elements present in the human body?
   A. Oxygen
   B. Carbon
   C. Nitrogen
   D. Iron

6. Atoms usually unite with each other to form larger chemical units called:
   A. Energy levels
   B. Mass
   C. Molecules
   D. Shells

7. Substances whose molecules have more than one element in them are called:
   A. Compounds
   B. Orbitals
   C. Elements
   D. Neutrons

True or False

For each of the following statements, write "T" in the answer blank if it is true. If the statement is false, circle the incorrect word(s) and write the correct word(s) in the answer blank.

_____ 8.   *Matter* is anything that occupies space and has mass.

_____ 9.   In the body, most chemicals are in the form of electrons.

_____ 10. At the core of each atom is a nucleus composed of positively charged protons and negatively charged neutrons.

_____ 11. Orbitals are arranged into *energy levels* depending on their distance from the nucleus.

_____ 12. The *formula* for a compound contains symbols that represent each element in the molecule.

▶ *If you had difficulty with this section, review page 24.*

CHEMICAL BONDING

Multiple Choice

Circle the correct answer.

13. Ionic bonds are chemical bonds formed by the:
    A. Sharing of electrons between atoms
    B. Donation of protons from one atom to another
    C. Donation of electrons from one atom to another
    D. Acceptance of protons from one atom to another

14. Molecules that form ions when dissolved in water are called:
    A. Covalent bonds
    B. Electrolytes
    C. Isotopes
    D. Ionic bonds

15. When atoms share electrons, a/an _____ forms.
    A. Covalent bond
    B. Electrolyte
    C. Ionic bond
    D. Isotope

16. Covalent bonds:
    A. Break apart easily in water
    B. Are not easily broken
    C. Donate electrons
    D. None of the above

17. An example of an ionic bond is:
    A. NaCl
    B. Ca
    C. O
    D. P

18. If a molecule "dissociates" in water, it:
    A. Has taken on additional ions
    B. Has eliminated ions
    C. Separates to form free ions
    D. Forms a covalent bond

▶ *If you had difficulty with this section, review pages 25-27.*

INORGANIC CHEMISTRY

Match each term with its corresponding description or definition.

_____ 19. A type of compound
_____ 20. Compound essential to life
_____ 21. Dissolves solutes
_____ 22. Water plus common salt
_____ 23. Reactants combine only after (H) and (O) atoms are removed
_____ 24. Combine to form a larger product
_____ 25. The reverse of dehydration synthesis
_____ 26. Yields energy for muscle contraction
_____ 27. Alkaline compound
_____ 28. A measure of the H+ concentration
_____ 29. Easily dissociates to form H+ ions
_____ 30. Dissociates very little

A. Aqueous solution
B. Water
C. ATP
D. Base
E. Solvent
F. pH
G. Dehydration synthesis
H. Inorganic
I. Weak acid
J. Hydrolysis
K. Strong acid
L. Reactants

▶ *If you had difficulty with this section, review pages 27-30.*

ORGANIC CHEMISTRY

Match each numbered term with its category. Write the corresponding letter in the blank.

A. Carbohydrate   B. Lipid   C. Protein   D. Nucleic acid

_____ 31.   Monosaccharide

_____ 32.   Triglyceride

_____ 33.   DNA

_____ 34.   Cholesterol

_____ 35.   Amino acid

_____ 36.   Glycogen

_____ 37.   Sucrose

_____ 38.   Phospholipid

_____ 39.   Contains C, O, H, and N

_____ 40.   RNA

▷ *If you had difficulty with this section, review pages 30-35.*

UNSCRAMBLE THE WORDS

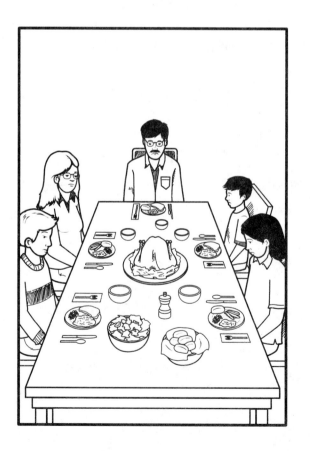

41. **N T E I P O R**

[ ][ ][ ](○)[ ][ ]

42. **S E B A**

[ ](○)[ ][ ]

43. **K L A L A N I E**

[ ][ ][ ](○)[ ][ ][ ]

44. **D L P I I**

[(○)][ ][ ][ ][ ]

Take the circled letters, unscramble them, and fill in the solution.

What was missing from the Thanksgiving dinner?

45. [ ][ ][ ][ ][ ]

Fill in the crossword puzzle.

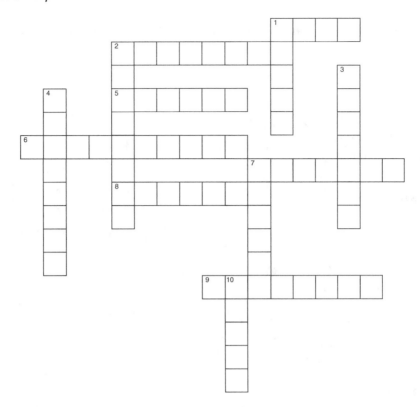

Across
1. Below 7.0 on pH scale
2. Bond formed by sharing electrons
5. Occupies space and has mass
6. Reverse of dehydration synthesis
7. Substances composed of one type of atom
8. Uncharged subatomic particle
9. Subatomic particle

Down
1. Combine to form molecules
2. Substances whose molecules have more than one element
3. Amino acid
4. Polysaccharide
7. Chemical catalyst
10. Fat

APPLYING WHAT YOU KNOW

46. Kim just finished preparing a meal of pan-fried hamburgers for her family. While the frying pan was still hot, she poured the liquid grease into a metal container to cool. Later, she noticed that the liquid oil had solidified as it cooled. Explain the chemistry of why the then room-temperature fat was solid.

47. Carol was gaining weight, yet she was eating very little. Her physician suspected hypothyroidism and suggested a test that measures radiation emitted by the thyroid when radioactive iodine is introduced into the gland. Describe what the radiologist will do to evaluate Carol's thyroid function.

48.   Word Find

Find and circle 12 terms presented in this chapter. Words may be spelled top to bottom, bottom to top, right to left, left to right, or diagonally.

Alkaline	Electrolyte
Atomic mass	Molecule
Base	Nucleic acid
Carbohydrate	Proton
Dehydration	Reactant
Dissociation	Solvent

E	T	A	R	D	Y	H	O	B	R	A	C	E
T	B	H	S	I	H	L	I	N	A	T	O	D
B	N	E	H	S	G	O	U	L	P	O	T	E
R	Z	A	M	S	F	R	K	U	S	M	T	H
P	R	O	T	O	N	A	I	E	C	I	X	Y
B	R	N	U	C	L	E	I	C	A	C	I	D
C	A	F	T	I	A	E	W	G	G	M	W	R
L	E	S	N	A	B	E	C	E	E	A	E	A
G	Q	E	E	T	E	A	R	U	S	S	F	T
Q	R	P	V	I	B	Y	K	I	L	S	W	I
E	T	Y	L	O	R	T	C	E	L	E	B	O
S	B	U	O	N	E	S	P	N	B	R	B	N
O	P	J	S	T	D	J	M	O	L	U	H	D

DID YOU KNOW?

After a vigorous workout, your triglycerides fall 10% to 20% and your HDL increases by the same percentage for 2 to 3 hours.

CHECK YOUR KNOWLEDGE

Fill in the blanks.

1. _____ is the field of science devoted to studying the chemical aspects of life.

2. Atoms are composed of protons, electrons, and _____.

3. The farther an orbital extends from the nucleus, the _____ its energy level.

4. Substances can be classified as _____ or _____.

5. Chemical bonds form to make atoms more _____.

6. A(n) _____ is an electrically charged atom.

7. Few _____ compounds have carbon atoms in them and none have C-C or C-H bonds.

8. _____ is a reaction in which water is lost from the reactants.

9. Chemists often use a _____ to represent a chemical reaction.

10. High levels of _____ in the blood make the blood more acidic.

11. _____ are compounds that produce an excess of H+ ions.

12. _____ maintain pH balance by preventing sudden changes in the H+ ion concentration.

13. _____ literally means "carbon" and "water."

14. _____ is a steroid lipid.

15. Collagen and keratin are examples of _____ proteins.

16. A _____ _____ _____ is formed when the twists and folds of the secondary structure fold again to form a three-dimensional structure.

17. A _____ _____ _____ is a sequence of amino acids in a chain.

18. In the DNA molecule, nucleotides are arranged in a twisted strand called a _____ _____.

19. RNA uses the same set of bases as DNA except for the substitution of _____ for thymine.

20. Glycogen and starch are examples of _____.

CHAPTER 3

Cells and Tissues

Cells are the smallest structural units of living things. Therefore, because we are living, we are made up of a mass of cells. Human cells, which vary in shape and size, can be seen only under a microscope. The three main parts of a cell are the cytoplasmic membrane, the cytoplasm, and the nucleus. As you review this chapter, you will be amazed at the correlation between a cell and the body as a whole. You will identify miniature circulatory systems, reproductive systems, digestive systems, power plants (much like muscular systems), and many other structures that will aid in your understanding of these body systems in future chapters.

Cells—just like humans—require water, food, gases, the elimination of wastes, and numerous other substances and processes in order to survive. The movement of these substances into and out of cells is accomplished by two primary methods: passive transport processes and active transport processes. In passive transport processes, no cellular energy is required to effect movement through the cell membrane. However, in active transport processes, cellular energy is required to provide movement through the cell membrane.

The study of cell reproduction completes this chapter's overview of cells. A basic explanation of DNA, "the hereditary molecule," illuminates the due respect for the amazing capability of the cell to transmit physical and mental traits from generation to generation. Reproduction of the cell—mitosis—is a complex process made up of several stages. These stages are outlined and diagrammed in the text to facilitate learning.

This chapter concludes with a discussion of tissues that reviews the four main types of tissues: epithelial, connective, muscle, and nervous. Knowledge of the characteristics, location, and function of these tissues is necessary to complete your understanding of this structural level of organization.

TOPICS FOR REVIEW

Before progressing to Chapter 4, you should have an understanding of the structure and function of the smallest living unit in the body—the cell. Your review should also include the methods by which substances move through the cell membrane and the stages that occur during cell reproduction. As you finish this chapter, you should have an understanding of tonicity and body tissues and the functions they perform in the body.

CELLS

Match each term on the left with its corresponding description on the right.

Group A

_A_ 1.	Cytoplasm	A. Component of plasma membrane
_E_ 2.	Plasma membrane	B. Controls reproduction of the cell
____ 3.	Cholesterol	C. "Living matter"
_B_ 4.	Nucleus	D. Paired organelles
____ 5.	Centrioles	E. Surrounds cells

Group B

_D_ 6.	Ribosomes	A. "Power plants"
E _D_ 7.	Endoplasmic reticulum	B. "Digestive bags"
_A_ 8.	Mitochondria	C. "Chemical processing and packaging center"
_B_ 9.	Lysosomes	D. "Protein factories"
C _E_ 10.	Golgi apparatus	E. "Smooth and rough"

Fill in the blanks.

11. The fat molecule ___Cholesterol___ helps stabilize the phospholipid molecules to prevent breakage of the plasma membrane.

12. A procedure performed prior to transplanting an organ from one individual to another is ___tissue___ ___typing___.

13. Fine, hairlike extensions found on the exposed or free surfaces of some cells are called ___cilia___.

14. Which organelle is distinguished by the fact that it has two types; it can be either smooth or rough. ___endoplasmic Reticulum___

15. ___ribosomes___ are usually attached to the rough endoplasmic reticulum and produce enzymes and other protein compounds.

16. The ___mitochondria___ provide energy-releasing chemical reactions that go on continuously.

17. The organelles that can digest and destroy microbes that invade the cell are called ___~~tysom~~ lysosomes___.

18. Mucus is an example of a product manufactured by the ___gulgi___ ___apparatus___.

19. Rod-shaped structures, known as ___~~chromosomes~~ centrioles___, play an important role during cell division.

20. ___chromatin___ ___granules___ are threadlike structures made up of proteins and DNA.

21. When the immune system mounts a significant attack against donated tissue, a ___organ rejection___ ___rejection reaction___ occurs.

22. The procedure used to test for the presence of antibodies produced in response to the HIV virus is known as _____.

▶ *If you had difficulty with this section, review pages 41-47 and page 67.*

MOVEMENT OF SUBSTANCES THROUGH CELL MEMBRANES

Circle the correct answer.

23. The energy required for active transport processes is obtained from:
    A. ATP
    B. DNA
    C. Diffusion
    D. Osmosis

24. An example of a passive transport process is:
    A. Permease system
    B. Phagocytosis
    C. Pinocytosis
    D. Diffusion

25. Movement of substances from a region of high concentration to a region of low concentration is known as:
    A. Active transport
    B. Passive transport
    C. Cellular energy
    D. Concentration gradient

26. Osmosis is the _____ of water across a selectively permeable membrane.
    A. Filtration
    B. Equilibrium
    C. Active transport
    D. Diffusion

27. _____ involves the movement of solutes across a selectively permeable membrane by the process of diffusion.
    A. Osmosis
    B. Filtration
    C. Dialysis
    D. Phagocytosis

28. A specialized example of diffusion is:
    A. Osmosis
    B. Permease system
    C. Filtration
    D. All of the above

29. Which movement always occurs down a hydrostatic pressure gradient?
    A. Osmosis
    B. Filtration
    C. Dialysis
    D. Facilitated diffusion

30. The uphill movement of a substance through a living cell membrane is:
    A. Osmosis
    B. Diffusion
    C. Active transport process
    D. Passive transport process

31. The ion pump is an example of what type of movement?
    A. Gravity
    B. Hydrostatic pressure
    C. Active transport process
    D. Passive transport process

32. An example of a cell capable of phagocytosis is the:
    A. White blood cell
    B. Red blood cell
    C. Muscle cell
    D. Bone cell

33. A salt solution that contains a higher concentration of salt than living red blood cells would be:
    A. Hypotonic
    B. Hypertonic
    C. Isotonic
    D. Homeostatic

34. A red blood cell becomes engorged with water and will eventually lyse, releasing hemoglobin into the solution. This solution is _____ to the red blood cell.
    A. Hypotonic
    B. Hypertonic
    C. Isotonic
    D. Homeostatic

 If you had difficulty with this section, review pages 47-53.

CELL REPRODUCTION AND HEREDITY

Circle the word in each word group that does not belong.

35. DNA	Adenine	Uracil	Thymine
36. Complementary base pairing	Guanine	RNA	Cytosine
37. Anaphase	Specific sequence	Gene	Base pairs
38. RNA	Ribose	Thymine	Uracil
39. Translation	Protein synthesis	mRNA	Interphase
40. Cleavage furrow	Anaphase	Prophase	2 daughter cells
41. Preparatory stage	Prophase	Interphase	DNA replication
42. Identical	Two nuclei	Telophase	Metaphase
43. Metaphase	Prophase	Telophase	Gene

 If you had difficulty with this section, review pages 53-59.

TISSUES

44. Fill in the missing areas of the chart.

TISSUE	LOCATION	FUNCTION
Epithelial		
1. Simple squamous	1a. Alveoli of lungs	1a. absorption
	1b. Lining of blood and lymphatic vessels	1b. Diffusion .
2. Stratified squamous	2a.	2a. Protection
	2b.	2b. Protection
3. Simple columnar	3.	3. Protection, secretion, absorption
4.	4. Urinary bladder	4. Protection
5. Pseudostratified	5.	5. Protection
6. Simple cuboidal	6. Glands; kidney tubules	6.

Connective		
1. Areolar	1.	1. Connection
2.	2. Under skin	2. Protection; insulation
3. Dense fibrous	3. Tendons; ligaments; fascia; scar tissue	3.
4. Bone	4.	4. Support, protection
5. Cartilage	5.	5. Firm but flexible support
6. Blood	6. Blood vessels	6.
7.	7. Red bone marrow	7. Blood cell formation
Muscle		
1. Skeletal (striated voluntary)	1.	1. Movement of bones
2. *cardiac*	2. Wall of heart	2. Contraction of heart
3. Smooth	3.	3. Movement of substances along ducts; change in diameter of pupils and shape of lens; "gooseflesh"
Nervous		
	1.	1. Irritability, conduction

▶ *If you had difficulty with this section, review Tables 3-7, 3-8, and 3-9 and pages 59-70.*

APPLYING WHAT YOU KNOW

45. Mr. Fee's boat capsized, and consequently he was stranded on a deserted shoreline for 2 days without food or water. When found, he had swallowed a great deal of seawater. He was taken to the emergency room in a state of dehydration. In the space below, draw the appearance of Mr. Fee's red blood cells as they would appear to the laboratory technician.

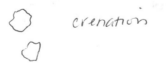
crenation

46. The nurse was instructed to dissolve a pill in a small amount of liquid medication. Just as she dropped the capsule into the liquid, she was interrupted by the telephone. On her return to the medication cart, she found the medication completely dissolved and apparently scattered evenly throughout the liquid. This phenomenon did not surprise her because she was aware from her knowledge of cell transport that _____*diffusion*_____ had created this distribution.

47. Ms. Bence has emphysema and has been admitted to the hospital unit with oxygen administered per nasal cannula. Emphysema destroys the tiny air sacs in the lungs. These tiny air sacs, alveoli, provide what function for Ms. Bence?   *gas exchange.*

48. Merrily was 5'4" and weighed 115 lbs. She appeared very healthy and fit, yet her doctor advised her that she was "overfat." What might be the explanation for this assessment?

49. Word Find

Find and circle 16 terms presented in this chapter. Words may be spelled top to bottom, bottom to top, right to left, left to right, or diagonally.

```
A  P  D  I  E  V  E  W  N  P  F  E  H  Y  X
I  G  I  Z  N  S  R  L  X  S  T  W  F  Z  S
R  J  V  N  N  T  A  I  L  M  R  P  H  M  F
D  W  U  E  O  O  E  H  B  E  A  D  U  G  F
N  W  I  U  I  C  I  R  P  O  N  N  F  B  W
O  P  U  R  S  H  Y  T  P  O  S  A  W  X  K
H  X  F  O  U  R  Y  T  A  H  L  O  G  A  W
C  L  Z  N  F  O  Y  P  O  R  A  E  M  R  M
O  U  I  X  F  M  L  F  O  S  T  S  T  E  O
T  T  B  Y  I  A  B  C  O  T  I  L  E  S  D
I  V  S  O  D  T  T  M  I  T  O  S  I  S  U
M  N  A  A  I  I  L  E  N  L  N  N  N  F  R
E  O  K  K  I  D  C  Q  H  B  I  V  I  T  H
E  K  T  X  B  Z  A  E  A  L  S  A  E  C  K
S  B  Z  R  P  M  V  L  X  W  Z  A  Z  C  V
```

Chromatid	Hypotonic	Pinocytosis
Cilia	Interphase	Ribosome
Cuboidal	Mitochondria	Telophase
DNA	Mitosis	Translation
Diffusion	Neuron	
Filtration	Organelle	

DID YOU KNOW?

The largest single cell in the human body is the female sex cell, the ovum. The smallest single cell in the human body is the male sex cell, the sperm.

CELLS AND TISSUES

Fill in the crossword puzzle.

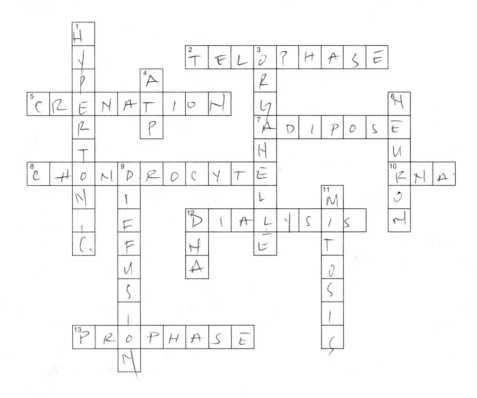

Across
2. Last stage of mitosis
5. Shriveling of cell due to water withdrawal
7. Fat
8. Cartilage cell
10. Ribonucleic acid (abbreviation)
12. Specialized example of diffusion
13. First stage of mitosis

Down
1. Having an osmotic pressure greater than that of the solution with which it is compared
3. Cell organ
4. Energy source for active transport
6. Nerve cell
9. Occurs when substances scatter themselves evenly throughout an available space
11. Reproduction process of most cells
12. Chemical "blueprint" of the body (abbreviation)

CHECK YOUR KNOWLEDGE

Multiple Choice

Circle the correct answer.

1. Which of the following cellular structures has the ability to secrete digestive enzymes?
   A. Lysosomes
   B. Mitochondria
   C. Golgi apparatus
   D. Ribosomes

2. Red blood cells do what when placed in a hypertonic salt solution?
   A. Remain unchanged
   B. Undergo crenation
   C. Lyse
   D. None of the above

3. Which of the following statements is true of chromatin granules?
   A. They exist in the cell cytoplasm.
   B. They are made up of DNA.
   C. They form spindle fibers.
   D. All of the above

4. In which stage of mitosis do chromosomes move to opposite ends of the cell along the spindle fibers?
   A. Anaphase
   B. Metaphase
   C. Prophase
   D. Telophase

5. Filtration is a process that involves which of the following?
   A. Active transport
   B. The expenditure of energy
   C. Changes in hydrostatic pressure
   D. All of the above

6. The synthesis of proteins by ribosomes using information coded in the mRNA molecule is called what?
   A. Translation
   B. Transcription
   C. Replication
   D. Crenation

7. Which of the following is *not* an example of connective tissue?
   A. Muscle
   B. Blood
   C. Fat
   D. Bone

8. Which of the following is the most abundant and widely distributed type of body tissue?
   A. Epithelial
   B. Connective
   C. Muscle
   D. Nerve

9. Simple, squamous epithelial tissue is made up of which of the following?
   A. A single layer of long, narrow cells
   B. Several layers of long, narrow cells
   C. A single layer of very thin and irregularly shaped cells
   D. Several layers of flat, scale-like cells

10. Which of the following groupings is correct when describing one of the muscle cell types?
    A. Visceral, striated, involuntary
    B. Skeletal, smooth, voluntary
    C. Cardiac, smooth, involuntary
    D. Skeletal, striated, voluntary

Matching

Match each term in column A with the most appropriate term in column B. (Only one answer is correct for each.)

Column A
____ F 11. Haversian system
____ G 12. Plasma membrane
____ J 13. Neuron
____ C 14. Pinocytosis
____ A 15. Prophase
____ B 16. Adenine
____ I 17. Diffusion
____ H 18. Squamous
____ D 19. Mitochondria
____ E 20. Visceral

Column B
A. Chromatids
B. Thymine
C. Active transport
D. Energy
E. Involuntary
F. Bone
G. Phospholipids
H. Flat
I. Passive transport
J. Axon

CELL STRUCTURE

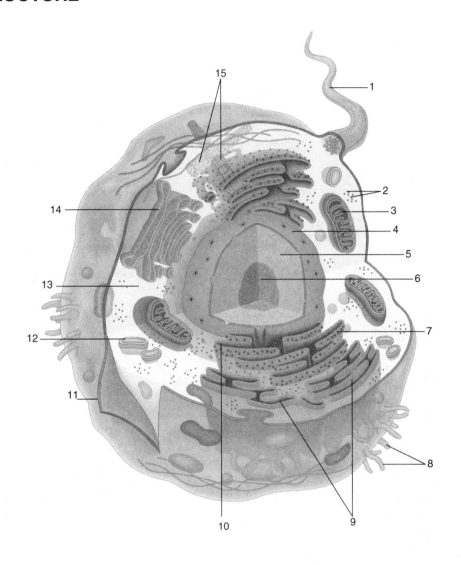

1. _____flagella_____
2. _____ribosomes_____
3. _____mitochondria_____
4. _____nuclear envelope_____
5. _____nucleus_____
6. _____nucleolus_____
7. _____endoplasmic reticulum_____
8. _____cilia_____
9. _____smooth_____
10. _____rough_____
11. _____plasma membrane_____
12. _____lysosomes_____
13. _____cytoplasm_____
14. _____golgi apparatus_____
15. _____centrioles_____

MITOSIS

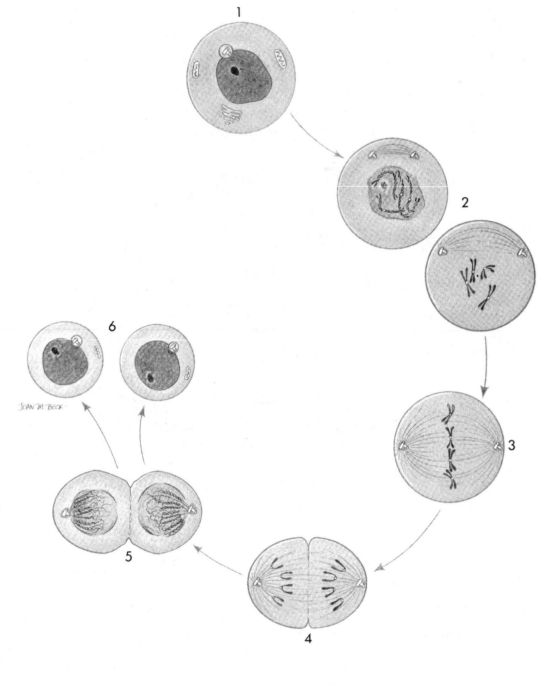

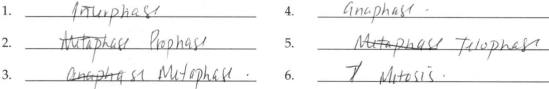

1. _____ Interphase _____   4. _____ Anaphase. _____

2. _____ Mitaphase Prophase _____   5. _____ Mitaphase Telophase _____

3. _____ Anaphase Mitaphase. _____   6. _____ T Mitosis. _____

TISSUES

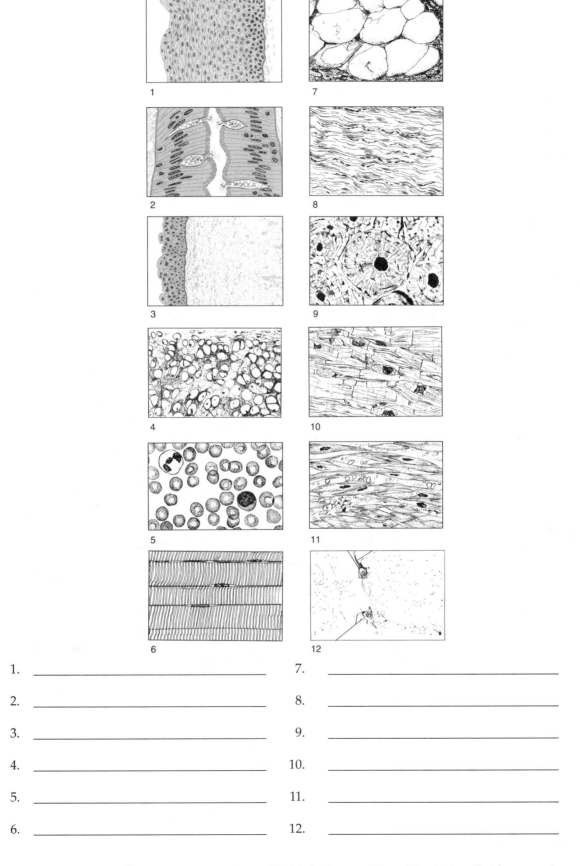

1. _____   7. _____

2. _____   8. _____

3. _____   9. _____

4. _____   10. _____

5. _____   11. _____

6. _____   12. _____

Organ Systems of the Body

A smooth-running automobile is the result of many systems working together harmoniously. The engine, the fuel system, the exhaust system, the brake system, and the cooling system are but a few of the many complex structural units that the automobile as a whole relies on to keep it functioning smoothly. So it is with the human body. We, too, depend on the successful performance of many individual systems working together to create and maintain a healthy human being.

When you have completed your review of the 11 major organ systems and the organs that make up these systems, you will find your understanding of the performance of the body as a whole much more meaningful.

TOPICS FOR REVIEW

Before progressing to Chapter 5, you should have an understanding of the 11 major organ systems and be able to identify the organs that are included in each system. Your review should also include current approaches to organ replacement.

ORGAN SYSTEMS OF THE BODY

Match each term on the left with its corresponding term on the right.

Group A

_____ 1.	Integumentary	A. Hair
_____ 2.	Skeletal	B. Spinal cord
_____ 3.	Muscular	C. Hormones
_____ 4.	Nervous	D. Tendons
_____ 5.	Endocrine	E. Joints

Group B

_____ 6.	Cardiovascular	A. Esophagus
_____ 7.	Lymphatic	B. Ureters
_____ 8.	Urinary	C. Larynx
_____ 9.	Digestive	D. Genitalia
_____ 10.	Respiratory	E. Spleen
_____ 11.	Reproductive	F. Capillaries

Circle the word in each word group that does not belong.

12. Pharynx	Trachea	Mouth	Alveoli
13. Uterus	Rectum	Gonads	Prostate
14. Veins	Arteries	Heart	Pancreas
15. Pineal	Bladder	Ureters	Urethra
16. Tendon	Smooth	Joints	Voluntary
17. Pituitary	Brain	Spinal cord	Nerves
18. Cartilage	Joints	Ligaments	Tendons
19. Hormones	Pituitary	Pancreas	Appendix
20. Thymus	Nails	Hair	Oil glands
21. Esophagus	Pharynx	Mouth	Trachea
22. Thymus	Spleen	Tonsils	Liver

23. Fill in the missing areas.

SYSTEM	ORGANS	FUNCTIONS
1. Integumentary	Skin, nails, hair, sense receptors, sweat glands, oil glands	
2. Skeletal		Support, movement, storage of minerals, blood formation
3. Muscular	Muscles	
4.	Brain, spinal cord, nerves	Communication, integration, control, recognition of sensory stimuli
5. Endocrine		Secretion of hormones; communication, integration, control
6. Cardiovascular	Heart, blood vessels	
7. Lymphatic		Transportation, immune system
8.	Kidneys, ureters, bladder, urethra	Elimination of wastes, electrolyte balance, acid-base balance, water balance
9. Digestive		Digestion of food, absorption of nutrients
10.	Nose, pharynx, larynx, trachea, bronchi, lungs	Exchange of gases in the lungs
11. Reproductive		Survival of species; production of sex cells, fertilization, development, birth; nourishment of offspring; production of hormones

▶ *If you had difficulty with this section, review pages 79-93 and the chapter summary on pages 97-99.*

ORGAN TRANSPLANTATION

Fill in the blanks.

24. An organ not required for life to continue is a _____
_____.

25. Many people suffering from deafness have had their hearing partially restored by "artificial ears" called _____ _____.

26. One of the earliest devices to augment vital functions was the "artificial kidney" or _____ _____.

27. Electromechanical devices that help keep blood pumping in patients suffering from end-stage heart disease are known as _____ _____ _____ _____.

28. One approach that offers the hope of a permanent solution to loss of vital organ function is _____ _____.

29. After cancerous breasts are removed, "new" breasts can be formed from skin and muscle tissue using a method known as _____ _____ _____.

30. The advantage to using a patient's own tissues in organ replacement is that the possibility of _____ is reduced.

▶ *If you had difficulty with this section, review pages 93-97.*

UNSCRAMBLE THE WORDS

31. **R T A H E**

[ ][ ][ ](O)[ ]

32. **I E P L N A**

[ ][ ](O)(O)[ ][ ]

33. **E E N V R**

[ ][ ][ ](O)[ ]

34. **S U H E S O P G A**

[ ](O)(O)[ ][ ][ ](O)[ ][ ]

Take the circled letters, unscramble them, and fill in the statement.

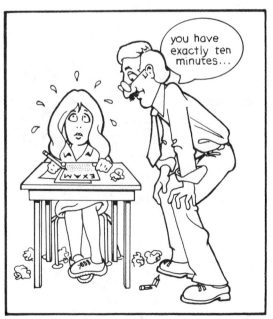

The more thoroughly you review this chapter, the less

35. [ ][ ][ ][ ][ ][ ][ ] **you will be during your test.**

APPLYING WHAT YOU KNOW

36. Myrna was 15 years old and had not yet started menstruating. Her family physician decided to consult two other physicians, each of whom specialized in a different system. Specialists in the areas of _____ and _____ were consulted.

37. Brian was admitted to the hospital with second- and third-degree burns over 50% of his body. He was placed in isolation. When Jenny went to visit him, she was required to wear a hospital gown and mask. Why was Brian placed in isolation? Why was Jenny required to wear special attire?

38. Sheila had a mastectomy to remove a cancerous lesion in her breast. Her body rejected the breast implant used to reconstruct her breast. Is there another breast reconstruction option that can be offered to Sheila? If so, explain this option.

39. Word Find

Find and circle the names of 11 organ systems. Words may be spelled top to bottom, bottom to top, right to left, left to right, or diagonally.

```
Y  R  A  T  N  E  M  U  G  E  T  N  I  R  F
H  N  E  R  V  O  U  S  K  I  R  J  M  G  T
L  Y  M  P  H  A  T  I  C  I  S  Y  Y  U  I
B  N  X  Y  R  O  T  A  L  U  C  R  I  C  W
P  E  L  R  E  O  M  J  M  S  O  M  M  P  S
C  C  W  M  A  N  D  L  A  T  E  L  E  K  S
R  R  K  E  M  L  I  U  A  A  V  V  U  K  N
D  K  X  P  D  J  U  R  C  J  I  R  Q  E  M
C  D  B  V  C  V  I  C  C  T  T  K  W  C  X
X  R  Q  Q  D  P  H  C  S  O  I  X  P  A  Z
M  F  M  U  S  Y  D  E  V  U  D  V  Y  K  E
U  E  S  E  C  Z  G  T  Q  D  M  N  E  K  O
P  Y  R  A  N  I  R  U  C  T  C  N  E  W  H
N  H  T  N  D  E  P  S  I  X  A  Q  O  I  E
```

Circulatory	Lymphatic	Respiratory
Digestive	Muscular	Skeletal
Endocrine	Nervous	Urinary
Integumentary	Reproductive	

DID YOU KNOW?

Muscles comprise 40% of your body weight. Your skeleton, however, only accounts for 18% of your body weight.

ORGAN SYSTEMS

Fill in the crossword puzzle.

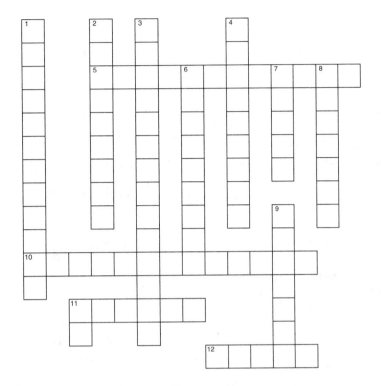

ACROSS

5. Specialized signal of nervous system (two words)
10. Skin
11. Testes and ovaries
12. Undigested residue of digestion

DOWN

1. Inflammation of the appendix
2. Vulva, penis, and scrotum
3. Heart and blood vessels
4. Subdivision of circulatory system
6. System of hormones
7. Waste product of kidneys
8. Agent that causes change in the activity of a structure
9. Chemical secretion of endocrine system
11. Gastrointestinal tract (abbreviation)

CHECK YOUR KNOWLEDGE

Multiple Choice

Circle the correct answer.

1. Which body system serves to clean the blood of waste products?
   A. Digestive
   B. Endocrine
   C. Cardiovascular
   D. Urinary

2. Ovaries and testes are considered components of which system?
   A. Reproductive system
   B. Endocrine system
   C. Both A and B
   D. None of the above

3. Which of the following organs is classified as an accessory organ of the digestive system?
   A. Mouth
   B. Esophagus
   C. Tongue
   D. Anal canal

4. Factors in the environment such as heat, light, pressure, and temperature that can be recognized by the nervous system are called:
   A. Effectors
   B. Stimuli
   C. Receptors
   D. Nerve impulses

5. Which body system stores the mineral calcium?
   A. Cardiovascular
   B. Digestive
   C. Lymphatic
   D. Skeletal

6. What is undigested material in the gastrointestinal tract called?
   A. Feces
   B. Urine
   C. Lymph
   D. Blood

7. Which body system produces heat and maintains body posture?
   A. Endocrine
   B. Muscular
   C. Cardiovascular
   D. Skeletal

8. Which of the following is *not* a function of the integumentary system?
   A. Integration
   B. Temperature regulation
   C. Ability to serve as a sense organ
   D. Protection

9. Which of the following is *not* a component of the digestive system?
   A. Spleen
   B. Liver
   C. Pancreas
   D. Gallbladder

10. When a group of tissues starts working together to perform a common function, what level of organization is achieved?
    A. Systemic
    B. Tissue
    C. Organ
    D. Cellular

Matching

Match each word in column A with the most appropriate corresponding word in column B. (There is only one correct answer for each.)

Column A

_____ 11. Sweat glands

_____ 12. Heart

_____ 13. Spleen

_____ 14. Vas deferens

_____ 15. Bladder

_____ 16. Gallbladder

_____ 17. Uterine tubes

_____ 18. Trachea

_____ 19. Spinal cord

_____ 20. Adrenals

Column B

A. Endocrine

B. Urinary

C. Integumentary

D. Cardiovascular

E. Respiratory

F. Digestive

G. Male reproductive

H. Lymphatic

I. Female reproductive

J. Nervous

CHAPTER 5

Mechanisms of Disease

One of our foremost concerns is health. We are fascinated and constantly confronted with information regarding what is necessary to be in good health, what is required for proper maintenance of the body, and what behaviors are responsible for disease.

Organisms play an important role in health. They are microscopic structures that are present everywhere. Many organisms are helpful and may be used in the preparation of foods, in industry and agriculture, in connection with solving the problems of how best to create shelter or clothing, and in combating disease. However, many other organisms are responsible for producing disease. They attack and disturb the normal homeostasis of the body and adversely affect our health. Many varieties of organisms exist. They are often classified by shape, size, function, or staining properties. To prevent disease, we must prevent pathogenic or disease-producing organisms from entering the body. This is not an easy task because we are surrounded by pathogenic organisms. It is important that we understand the transmission and control of these organisms to fully comprehend the mechanisms of disease.

TOPICS FOR REVIEW

Before progressing to Chapter 6 you should familiarize yourself with disease terminology and patterns of disease. You should continue your review by studying pathophysiology and pathogenic organisms. Finally, an understanding of tumors, cancer, and inflammation is necessary to round out your knowledge of this chapter.

STUDYING DISEASE

Match each term on the left with its corresponding description on the right.

Group A

___B___ 1. Pathology

___E___ 2. Signs A

___a___ 3. Symptoms E

___C___ 4. Syndrome C

___D___ 5. Etiology D

A. Subjective abnormalities

B. Study of disease

C. Collection of different signs and symptoms that present a clear picture of a pathological condition

D. Study of factors involved in causing a disease

E. Objective abnormalities

Group B

_C_ 6. Latent C   A. ~~Recovery~~

_a_ 7. Convalescence A   B. Disease native to a local region

_D_ 8. Pandemics P   C. ~~"Hidden"~~ stage

_B_ 9. Endemic B   D. ~~Epidem~~ics that spread throughout the world

_E_ 10. Pathogenesis E   E. Actual pattern of a disease's development

▶ *If you had difficulty with this section, review pages 103-105.*

PATHOPHYSIOLOGY

Fill in the blanks.

11. ___pathophysiology___ is the organized study of the underlying physiological processes associated with disease.

12. Many diseases are best understood as disturbances of ___homeostasis___.

13. Altered or ___mutated___ genes can cause abnormal proteins to be made.

14. An organism that lives in or on another organism to obtain its nutrients is called a ___parasite___.

15. Abnormal tissue growths may also be referred to as ___tumors___.

16. *Autoimmunity* literally means ___inflammation___.

17. Genetic factors, age, lifestyle, stress, environmental factors, and preexisting conditions are ___risk___ ___factors___ that may be responsible for predisposing a person to disease.

18. Scientists at the _____ _____ _____ _____ continuously track the incidence and spread of disease in this country and worldwide.

19. Conditions caused by psychological factors are sometimes called ___psychogenic___ disorders.

20. A primary condition can put a person at risk for developing a ___secondary___ condition.

▶ *If you had difficulty with this section, review pages 105-108.*

PATHOGENIC ORGANISMS

Circle the correct answer.

21. The smallest of all pathogens—microscopic nonliving particles—are called:
    A. Bacteria
    B. Fungi
    C. Viruses
    D. Protozoa

22. A tiny, primitive cell without a nucleus is called a:
    A. Bacterium
    B. Fungus
    C. Virus
    D. Protozoa

23. An example of a viral disease is:
    A. Diarrhea
    B. Mononucleosis
    C. Syphilis
    D. Toxic shock syndrome

24. Bacteria that require oxygen for metabolism are classified as:
    A. Gram positive
    B. Gram negative
    C. Aerobic
    D. Anaerobic

25. Bacilli are shaped like:
    A. Spheres
    B. Curves
    C. Squares
    D. Rods

26. Without chlorophyll, _____ cannot produce their own food, so they must consume or parasitize other organisms.
    A. Bacteria
    B. Fungi
    C. Viruses
    D. Protozoa

27. Protozoa include:
    A. Amoebas
    B. Flagellates
    C. Ciliates
    D. All of the above

28. Pathogenic animals include which of the following?
    A. Nematodes
    B. Platyhelminths
    C. Arthropods
    D. All of the above

29. The key to preventing diseases caused by pathogenic organisms is to:
    A. Have an annual physical
    B. Stop them from entering the body
    C. Isolate yourself from all disease-carrying individuals
    D. None of the above

30. The destruction of all living organisms is known as:
    A. Disinfection
    B. Antisepsis
    C. Sterilization
    D. Isolation

31. Ways in which pathogens can spread include:
    A. Person-to-person contact
    B. Environmental contact
    C. Opportunistic invasion
    D. Transmission by vector
    E. All of the above

32. Compounds produced by certain living organisms that kill or inhibit pathogens are:
    A. Antiseptics
    B. Antibiotics
    C. Disinfectants
    D. Sterilizers

▶ *If you had difficulty with this section, review pages 108-118.*

TUMORS AND CANCER

Circle the correct answer.

33. Benign tumors usually grow (*slowly* or *quickly*).

34. Malignant tumors (*are* or *are not*) encapsulated.

35. An example of a benign tumor that arises from epithelial tissue is (*papilloma* or *lipoma*).

36. A general term for malignant tumors that arise from connective tissues is (*melanoma* or *sarcoma*).

37. Abnormal, undifferentiated tumor cells are often produced by a process called (*hyperplasia* or *anaplasia*).

38. A cancer specialist is an (*osteologist* or *oncologist*).

39. The Papanicolaou test is a (*biopsy* or *MRI*).

40. (*Staging* or *Grading*) involves classifying a tumor based on its size and the extent of its spread.

41. Cachexia involves a loss of (*appetite* or *hair*).

▶ *If you had difficulty with this section, review pages 118-124.*

WARNING SIGNS OF CANCER

List the eight warning signs of cancer.

42. _____   46. _____

43. _____   47. _____

44. _____   48. _____

45. _____   49. _____

▶ *If you had difficulty with this section, review page 121.*

INFLAMMATION

If the statement is true, write "T" in the answer blank. If the statement is false, correct the statement by circling the incorrect term and writing the correct term in the answer blank.

_____T_____ 50. As tissue cells are damaged, they release inflammation mediators such as histamines, prostaglandins, and kinins.

_____F_____ 51. Inflammatory exudate is quickly removed by lymphatic vessels and carried to lymph nodes, which act as filters.

_____F_____ 52. Inflammation mediators can also act as signals that attract red blood cells to the injury site.

_____T_____ 53. The movement of white blood cells in response to chemical attractants is called *chemotaxis*.

_____T_____ 54. Inflammation can be local or systemic.

_____T_____ 55. Fevers usually subside after the irritant has been eliminated.

_____T_____ 56. The fever response in children and in older adults often differs from that in the normal adult.

▶ *If you had difficulty with this section, review pages 124-126.*

UNSCRAMBLE THE WORDS

57. **N G F U I**

f u [n] [g] i

58. **C E O N O G N E**

o [n] c o [g] e [n] e

59. **A D E E M**

a [d] e m [a]

60. **R S P O E**

s p o [r] [e]

Take the circled letters, unscramble them, and fill in the solution.

g i n g d a r

What Mr. Lynch found to be most difficult as a teacher.

61. g r a d i n g

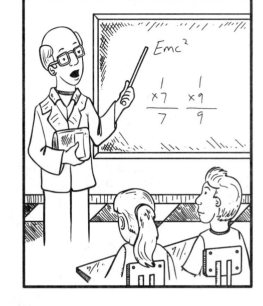

APPLYING WHAT YOU KNOW

62. Trent was examined by his doctor and was diagnosed as having a rhinovirus. Does he have need for concern? Why or why not?

63. Julius, a 2-year-old child, was experiencing rectal itching and insomnia. The pediatrician told Julius' mother that he suspected a nematode. What is the common term for the specific nematode that might cause these symptoms?

64. Shirley was cleaning her house and wanted to use the most appropriate and effective aseptic method to prevent the spread of germs. What would you suggest?

65. Mr. and Mrs. Gibbs adopted a child of Chinese descent. Mrs. Gibbs researched the "gene pool" of the child to alert her to any special concerns. What is a "gene pool" and how will this information assist Mr. and Mrs. Gibbs in the rearing of their child?

66. Bill has decided to become a paramedic. When he applied for school, it was suggested that he receive the series of vaccinations for hepatitis B. Why?

67. Word Find

Find and circle 18 terms presented in this chapter. Words may be spelled top to bottom, bottom to top, right to left, left to right, or diagonally.

```
N  P  E  S  D  B  S  L  A  A  C  E  R
W  O  L  S  I  C  I  M  E  D  I  P  E
X  V  I  O  F  S  X  V  R  E  N  A  T
O  D  P  T  U  E  A  D  O  N  C  R  U
H  S  O  V  A  S  T  T  P  O  U  A  C
Y  S  M  P  U  M  O  A  S  M  B  S  A
Y  P  A  R  O  I  M  B  I  A  A  I  I
N  L  I  O  S  R  E  A  F  L  T  T  D
W  V  J  T  C  Z  H  C  L  L  I  E  Y
W  Q  K  O  W  G  C  T  Q  F  O  C  M
V  Q  F  Z  I  F  G  E  R  P  N  F  A
K  E  N  O  Q  E  J  R  B  A  F  I  L
B  B  J  A  F  E  N  I  C  C  A  V  H
W  Z  F  H  R  B  S  U  D  M  Q  D  C
M  X  E  C  K  M  B  M  K  U  O  Z  P
```

Acute	Chlamydia	Metastasis
Adenoma	Ciliate	Parasite
Arthropod	Epidemic	Protozoa
Bacterium	Incubation	Spore
Biopsy	Inflammation	Vaccine
Chemotaxis	Lipoma	Virus

DID YOU KNOW?

As many as 500,000 Americans die from cancer each year, making it the second-leading cause of death after cardiovascular disease. Half of all cancers are diagnosed in people under the age of 67.

The hepatitis B virus (HBV) has infected more than 250 million people worldwide.

MECHANISMS OF DISEASE

Fill in the crossword puzzle.

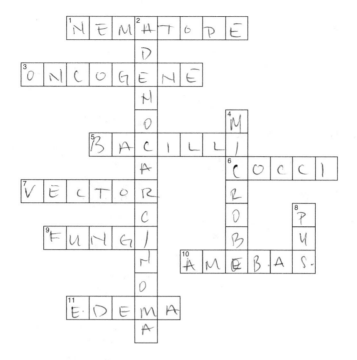

ACROSS

1. Roundworm
3. "Cancer gene"
5. Rod-shaped cells
6. Round cells
7. Spreads disease to other organisms
9. Lack chlorophyll
10. Possess pseudopodia
11. Tissue swelling

DOWN

2. Glandular cancer
4. Microscopic organism
8. Thick inflammatory exudate

CHECK YOUR KNOWLEDGE

Multiple Choice

Circle the correct answer.

1. Diseases with undetermined causes are:
   A. Asymptomatic
   B. Idiopathic
   C. Psychogenic
   D. Predisposing

2. The study of the occurrence, distribution, and transmission of diseases is:
   A. Entomology
   B. Pathology
   C. Oncology
   D. Epidemiology

3. Streptomycin is an example of a/an:
    A. Antibiotic
    B. Vaccine
    C. Pathogenic organism
    D. All of the above

4. Reversal of a chronic condition is called:
    A. Inflammatory response
    B. Predisposing condition
    C. Hemostasis
    D. Remission

5. If antibodies are found in an immunological test, it is assumed that:
    A. The patient has been exposed to a pathogen
    B. The infection is gone
    C. A and B
    D. None of the above

6. An epidemiologist:
    A. Studies the transmission of disease
    B. Monitors infection control programs
    C. Tracks the spread of disease
    D. All of the above

7. Study of the underlying physiological processes associated with disease leads to:
    A. Strategies of prevention
    B. Strategies of treatment
    C. A and B
    D. None of the above

8. Severe loss of appetite, weight loss, and general weakness in a cancer patient describe:
    A. Secondary infection
    B. Cachexia
    C. Inflammatory response
    D. Chemotaxis

9. Intracellular parasites that are not technically living organisms are characteristics of:
    A. Bacteria
    B. Fungi
    C. Amoebas
    D. Viruses

10. Examples of protozoa include all of the following *except*:
    A. Bacilli
    B. Flagellates
    C. Sporozoa
    D. Amoebas

Matching

Match each term in column A with the most appropriate definition or description in column B. (Only one answer is correct for each.)

Column A

___C___ 11. Syndrome

___D___ 12. Metastasis

___B___ 13. Anaerobic

___J___ 14. Protozoa

___G___ 15. Pathogenesis

___I___ 16. Fever

___E___ 17. Metazoa

___A___ 18. Pathology

___F___ 19. Neoplasm

___H___ 20. Arthropods

Column B

A. Study of disease

B. Require absence of oxygen

C. Collection of signs and symptoms

D. Spread of cancer cells

E. Multicellular organisms that parasitize humans

F. Abnormal cell growth

G. Pattern of disease development

H. Mites

I. Inflammatory response

J. One-celled organisms that parasitize cells

MAJOR GROUPS OF PATHOGENIC BACTERIA

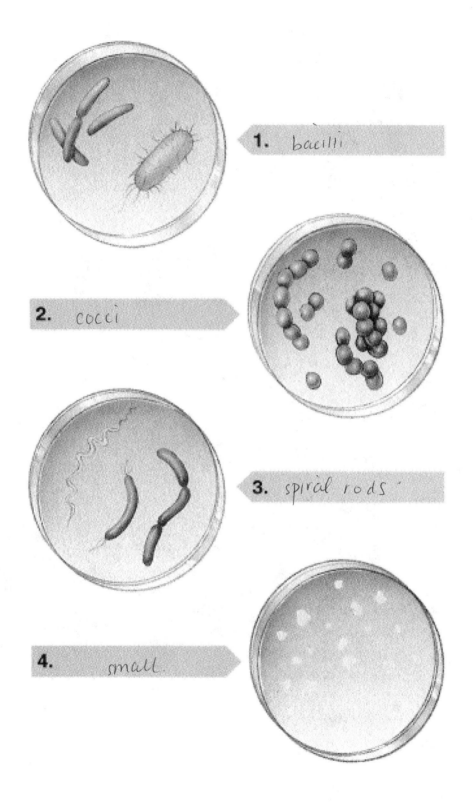

1. bacilli

2. cocci

3. spiral rods

4. small

MAJOR GROUPS OF PATHOGENIC PROTOZOA

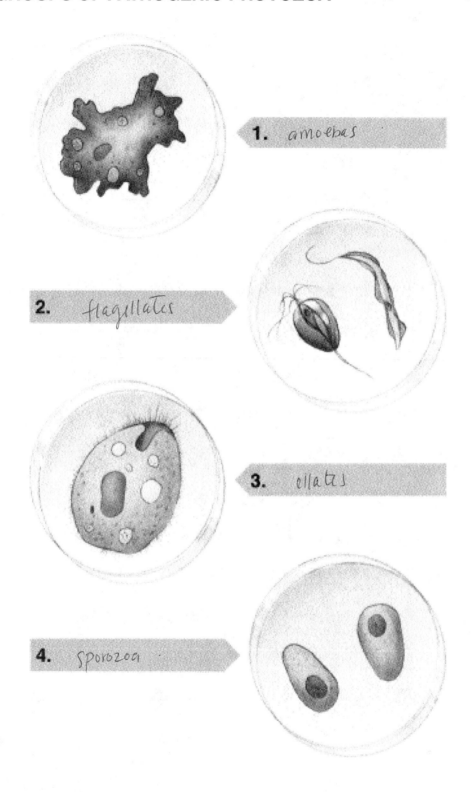

1. amoebas

2. flagellates

3. ciliates

4. sporozoa

EXAMPLES OF PATHOGENIC ANIMALS

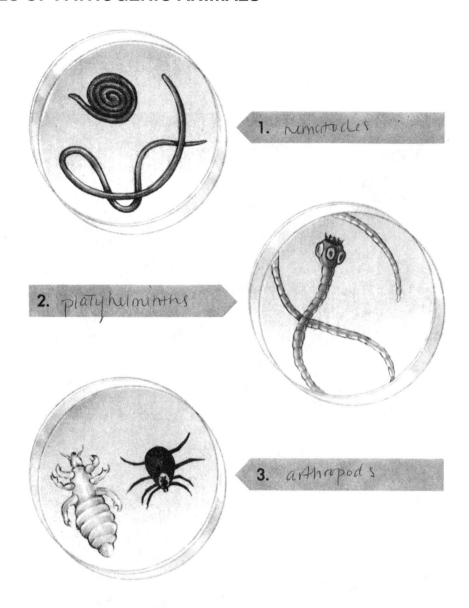

1. nematodes

2. platyhelminths

3. arthropods

MAJOR GROUPS OF PATHOGENIC FUNGI

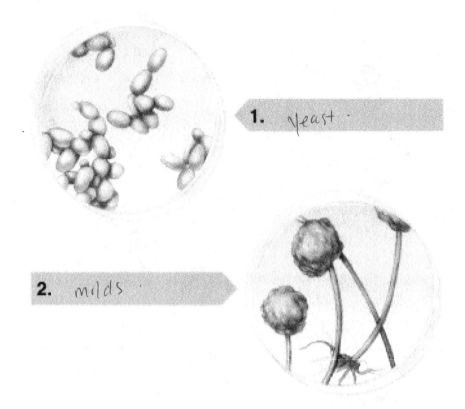

1. Yeast .

2. molds .

CHAPTER 6

The Integumentary System and Body Membranes

More of our time, attention, and money are spent on the integumentary system than on any other. Every time we look into a mirror we become aware of the integumentary system, as we observe our skin, hair, nails, and the appendages that give luster and comfort to this system. The discussion of the skin begins with the structure and function of the two primary layers called the *epidermis* and *dermis*. It continues with an examination of the appendages of the skin, which include the hair, receptors, nails, sebaceous glands, and sudoriferous glands. The study of skin concludes with a review of one of the most serious and frequent threats to the skin—burns. An understanding of the integumentary system provides you with an appreciation of the danger that severe burns could pose to this system.

Membranes are thin, sheetlike structures that cover, protect, anchor, or lubricate body surfaces, cavities, or organs. The two major categories of membranes are epithelial and connective. Each type is located in specific areas of the body and each is vulnerable to specific disease conditions. Knowledge of the location and function of these membranes prepares you for the study of their relationship to other systems and the body as a whole.

TOPICS FOR REVIEW

Before progressing to Chapter 7, you should have an understanding of the skin, its appendages, major skin disorders, and infections. Your review should include the classification of burns and the method used to estimate the percentage of body surface area affected by burns. A knowledge of the types of body membranes, their location, and their function is necessary to complete your study of this chapter.

CLASSIFICATION OF BODY MEMBRANES

Match each numbered term or description with its category and write the corresponding letter in the answer blank.

A. Cutaneous   B. Serous   C. Mucous   D. Synovial

_____ 1. Pleura

_____ 2. Lines joint spaces

_____ 3. Respiratory tract

_____ 4. Skin

_____ 5. Peritoneum

_____ 6. Contains no epithelium

_____ 7. Urinary tract

_____ 8. Lines body surfaces that open directly to the exterior

▶ *If you had difficulty with this section, review pages 133-135.*

THE SKIN

Match each term on the left with its description or definition on the right.

Group A

_____ 9. Integumentary system   A. Outermost layer of skin

_____ 10. Epidermis   B. Deeper of the two layers of skin

_____ 11. Dermis   C. Hypodermis

_____ 12. Subcutaneous   D. The skin is the primary organ

_____ 13. Cutaneous membrane   E. Composed of dermis and epidermis

Group B

_____ 14. Keratin   A. Protective protein

_____ 15. Melanin   B. Blue-gray color of skin resulting from a decrease in oxygen

_____ 16. Stratum corneum   C. Rows of peglike projections

_____ 17. Dermal papillae   D. Brown pigment

_____ 18. Cyanosis   E. Outer layer of epidermis

Match each numbered term or description with its corresponding skin layer and write A or B in the answer blank.

A. Epidermis   B. Dermis

_____ 19. Tightly packed epithelial cells

_____ 20. Nerves

_____ 21. Fingerprints

_____ 22. Blisters

_____ 23. Keratin

_____ 24. Connective tissue

_____ 25. Follicle

_____ 26. Sebaceous gland

_____ 27. Sweat gland

_____ 28. More cellular than the other layer

▶ *If you had difficulty with this section, review pages 133-144.*

Fill in the blanks.

29. The three most important functions of the skin are _____, _____, and _____.

30. _____ prevents the sun's ultraviolet rays from penetrating the interior of the body.

31. The hair of a newborn infant is called _____.

32. Hair growth begins from a small, cap-shaped cluster of cells called the _____ _____.

33. Hair loss of any kind is called _____.

34. The _____ _____ muscle produces "goose pimples."

35. A birthmark that appears as a bruise at birth and grows rapidly into a bright red nodule is called a _____ _____.

36. The most numerous, important, and widespread sweat glands in the body are the _____ sweat glands.

37. The _____ sweat glands are found primarily in the axilla and in the pigmented skin areas around the genitals.

38. _____ has been described as "nature's skin cream."

▶ *If you had difficulty with this section, review pages 137-144.*

Circle the correct answer.

39. A first-degree burn (*will* or *will not*) blister.

40. A second-degree burn (*will* or *will not*) scar.

41. A third-degree burn (*will* or *will not*) cause pain immediately.

42. According to the "rule of nines," the body is divided into (*9* or *11*) areas of 9% each.

43. Destruction of the subcutaneous layer occurs in (*second-* or *third-*) degree burns.

▶ *If you had difficulty with this section, review pages 147-149.*

DISORDERS OF THE SKIN

Circle the correct answer.

44. Any disorder of the skin may be called:
    A. Dermatitis
    B. Dermatosis
    C. Dermatotomy
    D. None of the above

45. Any measurable variation from the normal structure of a tissue is known as a/an:
    A. Lesion
    B. Burn
    C. Blister
    D. Erythema

46. An example of a papule is a:
    A. Scratch
    B. Bedsore
    C. Freckle
    D. Wart

47. An example of a skin disorder that may produce fissures is:
    A. Acne
    B. A bedsore
    C. Psoriasis
    D. Athlete's foot

48. The skin is the _____ line of defense against microbes that invade the body's internal environment.
    A. First
    B. Second
    C. Third
    D. Fourth

49. Tinea is a fungal infection and may appear as:
    A. Ringworm
    B. Jock itch
    C. Athlete's foot
    D. All of the above

50. Furuncles are local staphylococci infections and are also known as:
    A. Scabies
    B. Warts
    C. Boils
    D. Impetigo

51. The most common type of skin cancer is:
    A. Squamous cell
    B. Basal cell
    C. Melanoma
    D. Kaposi sarcoma

▶ *If you had difficulty with this section, review pages 146-152.*

UNSCRAMBLE THE WORDS

52. **P I D E E M I R S**

53. **R E K T A I N**

54. **A H I R**

55. **U G O N A L**

56. **D R T O N I D E H Y A**

Take the circled letters, unscramble
them, and fill in the solution.

What Amanda's mother gave her after every date.

57.

APPLYING WHAT YOU KNOW

58. Mr. Ziven was admitted to the hospital with second- and third-degree burns. Both arms, the anterior trunk, the right anterior leg, and the genital region were affected by the burns. The doctor quickly estimated that _____% of Mr. Ziven's body had been burned.

59. Mrs. James complained to her doctor that she had severe pain in her chest and feared that she was having a heart attack. An ECG revealed nothing unusual, but Mrs. James insisted that every time she took a breath she experienced pain. What might be the cause of Mrs. James' pain?

60. Mrs. Collins was born with a rare condition known as xeroderma pigmentosum. What activity should she avoid?

61. After investigating the scene of the crime, Officer Gorski announced that dermal papillae were found that would help solve the case. What did he mean?

62. Word Find

Find and circle 15 terms presented in this chapter. Words may be spelled top to bottom, bottom to top, right to left, left to right, or diagonally.

```
S  U  D  O  R  I  F  E  R  O  U  S  V  K  R
E  J  U  Q  U  E  S  T  E  C  N  O  H  Y  U
I  S  J  L  M  E  L  A  N  O  C  Y  T  E  H
R  I  M  U  E  N  O  T  I  R  E  P  H  S  B
O  M  K  N  V  A  S  T  R  L  A  N  U  G  O
T  R  G  U  F  G  A  U  C  E  G  O  V  W  D
A  E  A  L  P  R  D  I  O  N  T  F  D  R  N
L  D  V  A  D  M  L  C  P  D  H  S  L  Z  F
I  I  N  Y  N  L  R  L  A  M  E  N  I  R  E
P  P  H  Q  O  N  E  U  X  R  R  F  E  L  G
E  E  Z  F  J  U  M  Y  O  U  U  O  C  C  B
D  Z  P  E  R  J  Y  U  V  F  C  I  I  E  O
G  J  S  I  W  J  S  K  C  D  T  N  O  Z  C
C  O  S  M  Z  M  F  I  B  U  G  U  X  O  J
X  Y  P  M  E  I  W  E  C  V  S  U  G  B  I
```

Apocrine	Epidermis	Mucus
Blister	Follicle	Peritoneum
Cuticle	Lanugo	Pleurisy
Dehydration	Lunula	Serous
Depilatories	Melanocyte	Sudoriferous

DID YOU KNOW?

Because the dead cells of the epidermis are constantly being worn and washed away, we get a new outer skin layer every 27 days.

SKIN/BODY MEMBRANES

Fill in the crossword puzzle.

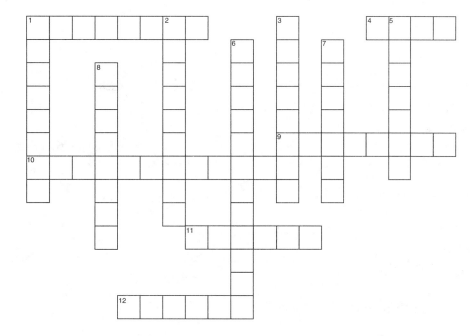

ACROSS

1. Inflammation of the serous membrane that lines the chest and covers the lungs
4. Cutaneous
9. Membrane that lines joint spaces
10. "Goose pimples" (two words)
11. Cushionlike sacs found between moving body parts
12. Deeper of the two primary skin layers

DOWN

1. Forms the lining of serous body cavities
2. Oil gland
3. Bluish-gray color of skin due to decreased oxygen
5. Tough waterproof substance that protects body from excess fluid loss
6. Sweat gland
7. Brown pigment
8. Covers the surface of organs found in serous body cavities

CHECK YOUR KNOWLEDGE

Multiple Choice

Circle the correct answer.

1. What type of serous membrane that covers organs is found in all body cavities?
   A. Visceral
   B. Pleural
   C. Parietal
   D. Synovial

2. Which of the following statements about synovial membranes is true?
   A. They are classified as epithelial.
   B. They line joints.
   C. They contain a parietal layer.
   D. All of the above are true.

3. Which of the following statements abut hair follicles is true?
   A. Arrector pili muscles are associated with them.
   B. Sudoriferous glands empty into them.
   C. They arise directly from the epidermis layer of skin.
   D. All of the above are true.

4. Which of the following statements about apocrine glands is true?
   A. They can be classified as sudoriferous.
   B. They are found primarily in armpit and genital regions.
   C. They secrete a thick substance that has a strong odor associated with it.
   D. All of the above are true.

5. Which of the following, if any, is *not* found in the dermis layer of the skin?
   A. Nerves
   B. Melanin
   C. Blood vessels
   D. All of the above are found in the dermis.

6. What characterizes second-degree burns?
   A. Blisters
   B. Swelling
   C. Severe pain
   D. All of the above

7. Blackheads can result from the blockage of which of the following glands?
   A. Lacrimal
   B. Sebaceous
   C. Ceruminous
   D. Sudoriferous

8. Keratin is found in which layer of the skin?
   A. Dermis
   B. Epidermis
   C. Subcutaneous
   D. Serous

9. What is the fold of skin that hides the root of a nail called?
   A. Lunula
   B. Body
   C. Cuticle
   D. Papillae

10. Which of the following is *not* an important function of the skin?
    A. Sense organ activity
    B. Absorption
    C. Protection
    D. Temperature regulation

Matching

Match each term in column A with its corresponding description in column B. (Only one answer is correct for each.)

Column A

_____ 11. Melanin

_____ 12. Epithelial membrane

_____ 13. Pacini corpuscle

_____ 14. Sebaceous

_____ 15. Waterproofing

_____ 16. Hair

_____ 17. Lunula

_____ 18. Connective tissue membrane

_____ 19. Dermal papillae

_____ 20. Sudoriferous

Column B

A. Fingerprint

B. Skin receptor

C. Brown pigment

D. Pleura

E. Synovial membrane

F. Perspiration

G. Oil

H. Follicle

I. Keratin

J. Little moon

Completion

Complete the following using the terms below. Write the corresponding letter in the answer blank.

A. Skin
B. Eccrine sweat glands
C. Peritonitis
D. Mucous

E. Epidermis
F. Fourth-degree burns
G. Pleurisy

H. Sebaceous
I. Hair follicles
J. Receptors

_____ 21. Which glands secrete oil or sebum for hair and skin?

_____ 22. The first line of defense for the body is the _____.

_____ 23. Which glands work throughout the body, helping to regulate body heat?

_____ 24. Which burn extends below the subcutaneous tissue to muscle or bone?

_____ 25. Hair growth requires epidermal, tubelike structures called _____.

_____ 26. The outermost and thinnest primary layer of skin is _____.

_____ 27. A condition that involves inflammation of the serous membranes lining the chest cavity and covering the lungs is called _____.

_____ 28. Which membrane lines body surfaces that open directly to the exterior of the body and produces mucus?

_____ 29. Specialized nerve endings that make it possible for skin to act as a sense organ are called _____.

_____ 30. An inflammation of the serous membranes lining the abdominal cavity and abdominal organs is called _____.

LONGITUDINAL SECTION OF THE SKIN

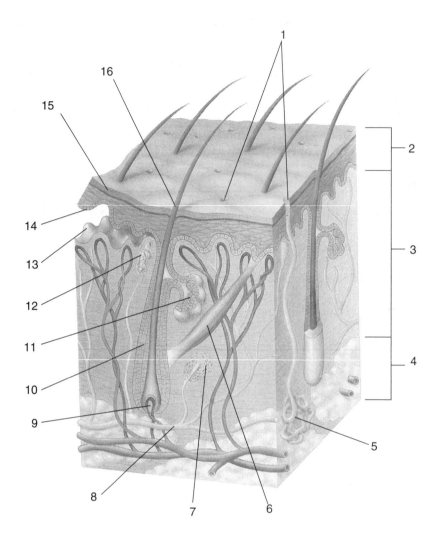

1. _____
2. _____
3. _____
4. _____
5. _____
6. _____
7. _____
8. _____

9. _____
10. _____
11. _____
12. _____
13. _____
14. _____
15. _____
16. _____

"RULE OF NINES" FOR ESTIMATING SKIN SURFACE BURNED

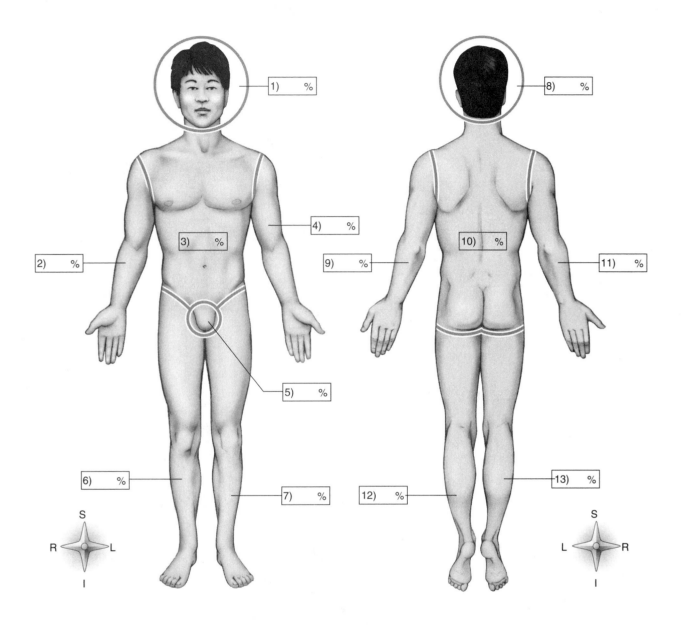

CHAPTER 7

The Skeletal System

How strange we would look without our skeleton! It is the skeleton that provides us with the rigid, supportive framework that gives shape to our bodies. But this is just the beginning, because the skeleton also protects the organs beneath it, maintains homeostasis of blood calcium, produces blood cells, and assists the muscular system in providing movement for us.

After reviewing the microscopic structure of bone and cartilage, you will understand how skeletal tissues are formed, their differences, and their importance in the human body. Your microscopic investigation will make the study of this system easier as you logically progress from this view to macroscopic bone formation and growth and visualize the structure of long bones.

The skeleton is divided into two main divisions: the axial skeleton and the appendicular skeleton. All of the 206 bones of the human body may be classified into one of these two areas. Although men and women have the same number and types of bones, subtle differences exist between a man's and a woman's skeleton. These structural differences provide us with insight into the functional differences between men and women.

Three types of joints exist in the body. They are classified according to the degree of movement they allow in the body. They are synarthroses, amphiarthroses, and diarthroses. It is important to have a knowledge of these joints to understand how movement is facilitated by articulations.

TOPICS FOR REVIEW

Before progressing to Chapter 8, you should familiarize yourself with the functions of the skeletal system, the structure and function of bone and cartilage, bone formation and growth, and the types of joints found in the body. Additionally, your understanding of the skeletal system should include identification of the two major subdivisions of the skeleton, the bones found in each area, and any differences that exist between a man's and a woman's skeleton. Your study should conclude with a review of the major skeletal disorders.

FUNCTIONS OF THE SKELETAL SYSTEM
TYPES OF BONES
STRUCTURE OF LONG BONES

Fill in the blanks.

1. There are _four : long short flat irregular_ types of bones.

2. The ___Medullary___ ___cavity___ is the hollow area inside the diaphysis of a bone.

3. A thin layer of cartilage covering each epiphysis is the ___articular___ ___cartlage___.

4. The ___endosteum___ lines the medullary cavity of long bones.

5. ___Hematapousis___ is used to describe the process of blood cell formation.

6. Blood cell formation is a vital process carried on in ___red bone marrow___ _____.

7. The ___periostem periosteum___ is a strong fibrous membrane that covers a long bone everywhere except at joint surfaces.

8. Bones may be classified by shape. Those shapes include ___long___, ___short___, ___flat___, and ___irregular___.

9. Bones serve as a safety-deposit box for ___calcium___, a vital substance required for normal nerve and muscle function.

10. As muscles contract and shorten, they pull on bones and thereby ___move___ them.

▷ *If you had difficulty with this section, review pages 163-165.*

MICROSCOPIC STRUCTURE OF BONE AND CARTILAGE

Match each term on the left with its corresponding description on the right.

Group A

_D_ 11.	Trabeculae	A. Outer covering of bone
_B_ 12.	Compact	B. Dense bone tissue
_E_ 13.	Spongy	C. Fibers embedded in a firm gel
_A_ 14.	Periosteum	D. Needle-like threads of spongy bone
_C_ 15.	Cartilage	E. Ends of long bones

Group B

_D_ 16.	Osteocytes	A. Connect lacunae
_A_ 17.	Canaliculi	B. Cartilage cells
_E_ 18.	Lamellae	C. Structural unit of compact bone
_B_ 19.	Chondrocytes	D. Bone cells
_C_ 20.	Haversian system	E. Ring of bone

▷ *If you had difficulty with this section, review pages 165-168.*

BONE FORMATION AND GROWTH

If the statement is true, write "T" in the answer blank. If the statement is false, correct the statement by circling the incorrect term and writing the correct term in the answer blank.

_____T_____ 21. When the skeleton forms in a baby before birth, it consists of cartilage and fibrous structures.

_____F_____ 22. The diaphyses are the ends of the bone.

_____F_____ 23. Bone-forming cells are known as *osteoclasts*.

_____T_____ 24. It is the combined action of osteoblasts and osteoclasts that sculpts bones into their adult shapes.

_____T_____ 25. The point of articulation between the epiphysis and diaphysis of a growing long bone is susceptible to injury if over-stressed.

_____F_____ 26. The epiphyseal plate can be seen in both external and cutaway views of an adult long bone.

_____F_____ 27. The shaft of a long bone is known as the *articulation*.

_____T_____ 28. Cartilage in the newborn becomes bone when it is replaced with calcified bone matrix deposited by osteoblasts.

_____F_____ 29. When epiphyseal cartilage becomes bone, growth begins.

_____T_____ 30. The epiphyseal cartilage is visible, if present, on x-ray films.

▶ *If you had difficulty with this section, review pages 168-170.*

DIVISIONS OF SKELETON

Circle the correct answer.

31. Which of the following is/are *not* a part of the axial skeleton?
    A. Scapula
    B. Cranial bones
    C. Vertebra
    D. Ribs
    E. Sternum

32. Which one of the following is *not* a cranial bone?
    A. Frontal
    B. Parietal
    C. Occipital
    D. Lacrimal
    E. Sphenoid

33. Which of the following is *not* correct?
    A. A baby is born with a straight spine.
    B. In the adult, the sacral and thoracic curves are convex.
    C. The normal curves of the adult spine provide greater strength than a straight spine.
    D. A curved structure has more strength than a straight one of the same size and materials.

34. True ribs:
    A. Attach to the cartilage of other ribs
    B. Do not attach to the sternum
    C. Attach directly to the sternum without cartilage
    D. Attach directly to the sternum by means of cartilage

35. The bone that runs along the lateral side of your forearm is the:
    A. Humerus
    B. Ulna
    C. Radius
    D. Tibia

36. The shinbone is also known as the:
    A. Fibula
    B. Femur
    C. Tibia
    D. Ulna

37. The bones in the palm of the hand are called:
    A. Metatarsals
    B. Tarsals
    C. Carpals
    D. Metacarpals

38. Which one of the following is *not* a bone of the upper extremity?
    A. Radius
    B. Clavicle
    C. Humerus
    D. Ilium

39. The heel bone is known as the:
    A. Calcaneus
    B. Talus
    C. Metatarsal
    D. Phalanges

40. The mastoid process is part of which bone?
    A. Parietal
    B. Temporal
    C. Occipital
    D. Frontal

41. When a baby learns to walk, which area of the spine becomes concave?
    A. Lumbar
    B. Thoracic
    C. Cervical
    D. Coccyx

42. Which bone is the "funny" bone?
    A. Radius
    B. Ulna
    C. Humerus
    D. Carpal

43. There are how many pair of true ribs?
    A. 14
    B. 7
    C. 5
    D. 3

44. The 27 bones in the wrist and the hand allow for more:
    A. Strength
    B. Dexterity
    C. Protection
    D. Red blood cell products

45. The longest bone in the body is the:
    A. Tibia
    B. Fibula
    C. Femur
    D. Humerus

46. Distally, the _____ articulates with the patella.
    A. Femur
    B. Fibula
    C. Tibia
    D. Humerus

47. Which bones form the cheek bones?
    A. Mandible
    B. Palatine
    C. Maxillary
    D. Zygomatic

48. In a child, there are five of these bones. In an adult, they are fused into one.
    A. Pelvic
    B. Lumbar vertebrae
    C. Sacrum
    D. Carpals

49. The spinal cord enters the cranium through a large hole (foramen magnum) in which bone?
    A. Temporal
    B. Parietal
    C. Occipital
    D. Sphenoid

Circle the word in each word group that does not belong.

50. Cervical	Thoracic	Coxal	Coccyx
51. Pelvic girdle	Ankle	Wrist	Axial
52. Frontal	Occipital	(Maxilla)	Sphenoid
53. Scapula	(Pectoral girdle)	Ribs	Clavicle
54. Malleus	(Vomer)	Incus	Stapes
55. (Ulna)	Ilium	Ischium	Pubis
56. Carpal	Phalanges	Metacarpal	(Ethmoid)
57. Ethmoid	Parietal	Occipital	(Nasal)
58. Anvil	Atlas	Axis	(Cervical)

▶ *If you have had difficulty with this section, review pages 170-184.*

DIFFERENCES BETWEEN A MAN'S AND A WOMAN'S SKELETON

Identify each skeletal structure as being typically male or female.

A. Male   B. Female

_____ 59.   Funnel-shaped pelvis

_____ 60.   Broader-shaped pelvis

__F__ 61.   Wider pubic angle

_____ 62.   Larger coxal bones

_____ 63.   Wider pelvic inlet

▶ *If you had difficulty with this section, review page 184.*

BONE MARKINGS

From the choices given, match each bone with its identification marking. Answer choices may be used more than once.

A. Mastoid
B. Pterygoid process
C. Foramen magnum
D. Sella turcica
E. Mental foramen
F. Conchae
G. Xiphoid process

H. Glenoid cavity
I. Olecranon process
J. Ischium
K. Acetabulum
L. Symphysis pubis
M. Ilium
N. Greater trochanter

O. Medial malleolus
P. Calcaneus
Q. Acromion process
R. Frontal sinuses
S. Condyloid process
T. Tibial tuberosity

_____ 64. Occipital

_____ 65. Sternum

_____ 66. Coxal

_____ 67. Femur

_____ 68. Ulna

_____ 69. Temporal

_____ 70. Tarsals

_____ 71. Sphenoid

_____ 72. Ethmoid

_____ 73. Scapula

_____ 74. Tibia

_____ 75. Frontal

_____ 76. Mandible

▶ *If you had difficulty with this section, review pages 172-182.*

JOINTS (ARTICULATIONS)

Circle the correct answer.

77. Freely movable joints are (*amphiarthroses* or *diarthroses*).

78. The sutures in the skull are (*synarthrotic* or *amphiarthrotic*) joints.

79. All (*diarthrotic* or *amphiarthrotic*) joints have a joint capsule, a joint cavity, and a layer of cartilage over the ends of the two joining bones.

80. (*Ligaments* or *Tendons*) grow out of periosteum and attach two bones together.

81. The (*articular cartilage* or *epiphyseal cartilage*) absorbs jolts.

82. Gliding joints are the (*least movable* or *most movable*) of the diarthrotic joints.

83. The knee is the (*largest* or *smallest*) joint.

84. Hinge joints allow motion in (*2* or *4*) directions.

85. The saddle joint at the base of each of our thumbs allows for greater (*strength* or *mobility*).

86. When you rotate your head, you are using a (*gliding* or *pivot*) joint.

▶ *If you had difficulty with this section, review pages 185-191.*

SKELETAL DISORDERS

Fill in the blanks.

87. _____arthroscopy._____ is an imaging technique that allows a physician to examine the internal structure of a joint without the use of extensive surgery.

88. One of the most common skeletal tumors and one of the most rapidly fatal is
_____osteosarcoma_____.

89. A common bone disease characterized by excessive loss of calcified matrix and collagenous fiber is
_____osteoporosis_____.

90. A metabolic disorder involving mineral loss in bones is _____.

91. A metabolic disorder that is often asymptomatic and affects older adults is
_____

92. The general name for bacterial infections of bone and marrow tissue is
_____osteomyelitis·_____.

93. Closed fractures, also known as _____simple_____
_____, do not pierce the skin.

94. _____ _____ are breaks that produce many fragments.

95. The most common noninflammatory joint disease is _____osteoarthritis_____ or
_____degenerative_____, _____joint_____
_____.

96. Three major types of arthritis are _____Rheumatoid_____,
_____Gouty·_____, and _____.

97. One form of infectious arthritis, _____
_____, was identified in 1975 in Connecticut and has since spread
across the continent.

▶ *If you had difficulty with this section, review pages 191-200.*

UNSCRAMBLE THE BONES

98. **E T V E R R B A E**

Ⓥ E T E Ⓑ Ⓡ Ⓐ A E

99. **B P S U I**

◯ ◻ ◯ ◻

100. **S C A L U P A**

S Ⓒ A P Ⓤ Ⓞ A

101. **I M D B A L N E**

◻ ◻ ◻ ◯ ◯ ◻ ◯

102. **A P N H G A E L S**

P H A Ⓞ A N Ⓖ E S

Take the circled letters, unscramble
them, and fill in the solution.

What the fat lady wore to the ball.

103. ◻◻◻◻◻◻   ◻◻◻◻◻◻

APPLYING WHAT YOU KNOW

104. Mrs. Perine had advanced cancer of the bone. As the disease progressed, Mrs. Perine required several blood transfusions throughout the time she was receiving therapy. She asked the doctor one day to explain the necessity for the transfusions. What explanation might the doctor give to Mrs. Perine?

105. Dr. Kennedy, an orthopedic surgeon, called the admissions office of the hospital and advised that he would be admitting a patient in the next hour with an epiphyseal fracture. Without any other information, the patient is assigned to the pediatric ward. What prompted this assignment?

106. Mrs. Van Skiver, age 75, noticed when she went in for her physical examination that she was a half inch shorter than she was on her last visit. Dr. Veazey suggested she begin a regimen of dietary supplements of calcium, vitamin D, and a prescription for sex hormone therapy. What bone disease did Dr. Veazey suspect?

107. Mr. Ferber was moving and experienced severe sharp pain in his lower back while lifting some boxes. The pain was not relieved by traditional home remedies or pain medication. He finally sought the advice of a physician after being unable to relieve the pain for 48 hours. What might be a possible diagnosis?

108. Word Find

Find and circle 13 terms presented in this chapter. Words may be spelled top to bottom, bottom to top, right to left, left to right, or diagonally.

```
S  A  N  A  R  T  I  C  U  L  A  T  I  O  N
I  O  M  P  L  T  C  A  P  M  O  C  E  S  C
M  H  E  P  T  T  A  M  A  S  A  I  A  T  P
O  E  L  F  H  T  A  E  P  N  I  F  L  E  T
S  M  L  A  S  I  E  I  A  O  O  P  U  O  S
S  A  M  O  I  L  A  L  O  N  I  E  C  B  T
E  T  S  U  N  X  I  R  T  R  A  T  E  L  S
S  O  B  T  E  C  A  A  T  N  A  E  B  A  A
R  P  I  E  U  T  N  E  U  H  O  O  A  S  L
S  O  T  L  C  E  S  C  T  A  R  S  R  T  C
U  I  I  R  L  O  A  O  O  O  A  O  T  S  O
N  E  T  S  H  L  T  A  I  R  I  I  S  A  E
I  S  T  H  E  U  O  A  M  R  C  X  S  E  T
S  I  S  T  A  I  E  T  C  R  E  S  I  A  S
L  S  C  A  S  H  S  T  O  I  O  P  T  S  O
```

Amphiarthroses	Fontanels	Osteoclasts
Articulation	Hematopoiesis	Periosteum
Axial	Lacunae	Sinus
Canaliculi	Osteoblasts	Trabeculae
Compact		

DID YOU KNOW?

The bones of the hands and feet make up more than half of the total 206 bones of the body.

Approximately 25 million Americans have osteoporosis. Four out of five are women.

The bones of the middle ear are mature at birth.

SKELETAL SYSTEM

Fill in the crossword puzzle.

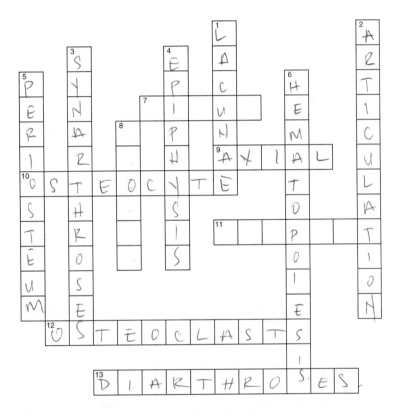

ACROSS	DOWN
7. Space inside cranial bone	1. Spaces in bones where osteocytes are found
9. Division of skeleton	2. Joint
10. Bone cell	3. Suture joints
11. Type of bone	4. Ends of long bones
12. Bone-absorbing cells	5. Covers long bone except at its joint surfaces
13. Freely movable joints	6. Process of blood cell formation
	8. Chest

CHECK YOUR KNOWLEDGE

Multiple Choice

Circle the correct answer.

1. Which of the following statements concerning the ribs is true?
   A. The first seven pairs attach to the sternum by cartilage.
   B. The last four pairs are called *floating ribs* because they are free in the front.
   C. The eighth, ninth, and tenth pairs do not move because they are not attached to the sternum.
   D. All of the above statements concerning the ribs are true.

2. Which is the largest bone in the lower extremities?
   A. Humerus
   B. Ulna
   C. Femur
   D. Radius

3. Of what is yellow bone marrow primarily made?
   A. Fatty tissue
   B. Blood cells
   C. Epithelial tissue
   D. Fibrous tissue

4. Which of the following statements regarding the female pelvis is *not* true?
   A. Its shape can be described as broader, shallower, and basinlike when compared to that of the male.
   B. Its pelvic inlet, or brim, is usually wider than that of the male.
   C. Its individual hipbones are usually larger and heavier than those of the male.
   D. All of the above statements are true.

5. Which of the following statements are true about the normal curves of the spine (two concave and two convex)?
   A. They are present at birth.
   B. They extend from the skull to the bottom of the ribcage.
   C. They give the spine strength to support the weight of the rest of the body.
   D. All of the above are true.

6. Which of the following statements regarding diarthrotic joints is *not* true?
   A. They contain a synovial membrane that secretes a lubricating fluid called *synovial fluid*.
   B. Diarthrotic joints may permit flexion, extension, abduction, adduction, or rotation.
   C. These joints make up the largest category of body joints.
   D. All of the above statements are true.

7. Which of the following bones are components of the axial skeletal system?
   A. Ilium, ethmoid, clavicle
   B. Ulna, palatine, occipital
   C. Sacrum, vomer, sphenoid
   D. Scapula, patella, fibula

8. Which of the following bones is *not* classified as a cranial bone?
   A. Sphenoid
   B. Parietal
   C. Palatine
   D. Temporal

9. Which of the following statements characterizes the skeleton of a growing child?
   A. Epiphyses are separated from diaphyses by a layer of cartilage.
   B. Osteoblasts deposit calcium in the gel-like matrix of cartilage.
   C. The periosteum is present.
   D. All of the above statements characterize the skeleton of a growing child.

10. What are the joints between the cranial bones called?
    A. Synarthroses
    B. Diarthroses
    C. Amphiarthroses
    D. All of the above

Matching

Match each term in column A with its corresponding description in column B. (Only one answer is correct for each.)

Column A

_____ 11. Diarthroses

_____ 12. Spongy bone

_____ 13. Synarthrosis

_____ 14. Foramen magnum

_____ 15. Calcaneus

_#_ 16. Chondrocyte

_____ 17. Compact bone

_____ 18. Ethmoid

_____ 19. Coxal

_____ 20. Hematopoiesis

Column B

A. Haversian canal

B. Trabeculae

C. Perpendicular plate

D. Red bone marrow

E. Tarsal

F. Ilium

G. Synovial fluid

H. Cartilage

I. Suture

J. Occipital bone

LONGITUDINAL SECTION OF LONG BONE

1. *articular cartilage*

2. *epiphyseal line*

3. *cancellous bone*

4. *red bone marrow spaces*

5. *compact bone*

6. *yellow bone marrow*

7. *periosteum*

8. *endosteum*

9. *Medullary cavity*

10. *epiphysis*

11. *diaphysis*

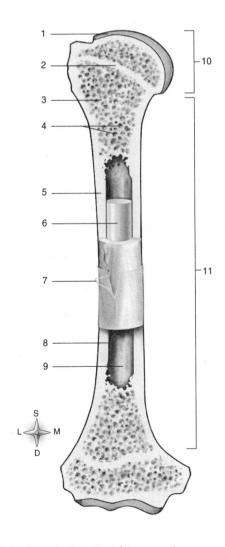

ANTERIOR VIEW OF SKELETON

1. ___Skull___
2. _____
3. ___Zygomatic___
4. ___Sternum___
5. _____
6. ___thoracic___
7. ___Ilium___
8. ___Pubis___
9. ___Ischium___
10. ___greater trochanter___
11. ___phalanges___
12. ___metatarsals___
13. ___tarsals___
14. _____
15. _____
16. ___patella___
17. ___femur___
18. ___phalanges___
19. ___metacarpals___
20. ___carpals___
21. ___ulna___
22. ___radius___
23. ___humerus___
24. ___xiphoid process___
25. _____
26. ___scapula___
27. _____
28. ___clavicle___
29. ___mandible___
30. _____

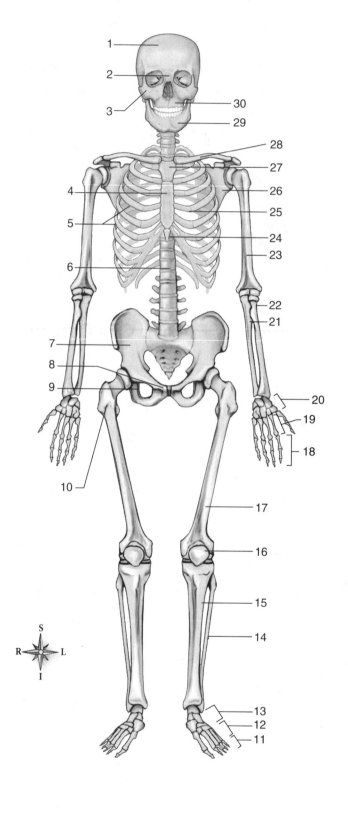

POSTERIOR VIEW OF SKELETON

1. ~~parietal~~
2. _____
3. _____
4. _____
5. _____
6. _____
7. _____
8. _____
9. _____
10. _____
11. _____
12. _____
13. _____
14. _____
15. _____
16. _____
17. _____
18. _____
19. _____
20. _____
21. _____
22. _____
23. lumbar
24. thoracic
25. cervical
26. _____
27. _____

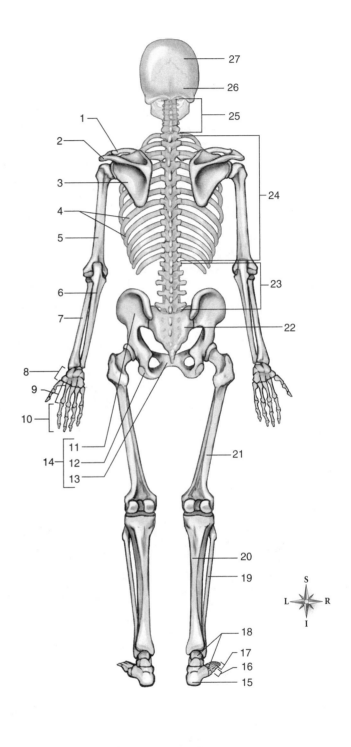

SKULL VIEWED FROM THE RIGHT SIDE

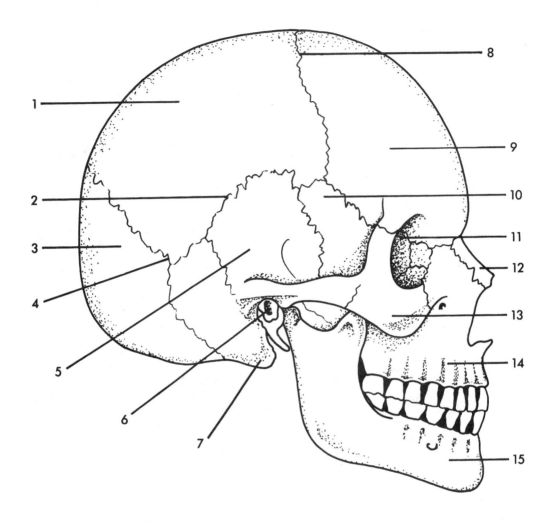

1. _____   9. _____

2. _____   10. _____

3. _____   11. _____

4. _____   12. _____

5. _____   13. _____

6. _____   14. _____

7. _____   15. _____

8. _____

SKULL VIEWED FROM THE FRONT

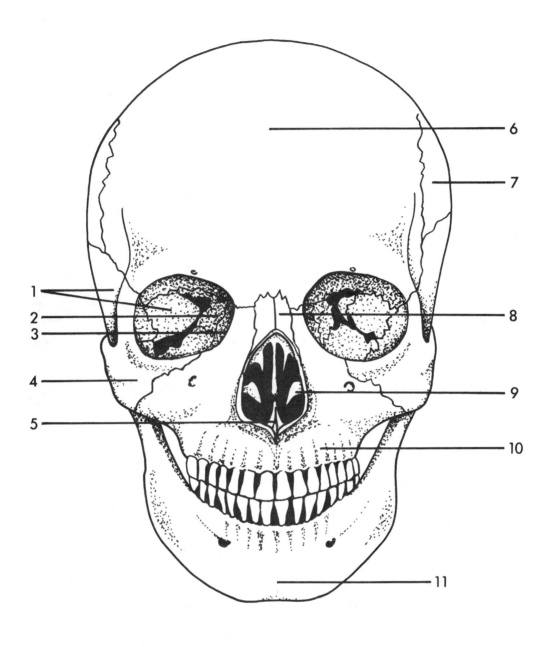

1. _____

2. _____

3. _____

4. _____

5. _____

6. _____

7. _____

8. _____

9. _____

10. _____

11. _____

STRUCTURE OF A DIARTHROTIC JOINT

1. _____

2. _____

3. _____

4. _____

5. _____

6. _____

7. _____

8. _____

9. _____

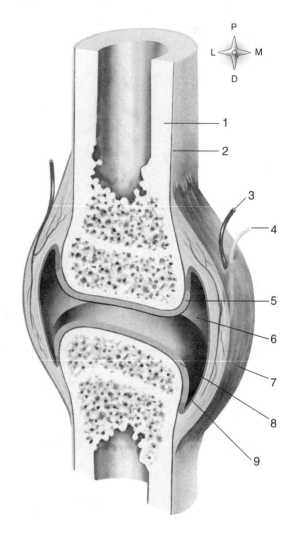

CHAPTER 8

The Muscular System

The muscular system is often referred to as the "power system," and rightfully so, because it is this system that provides the force necessary to move the body and perform many organ functions. Just as an automobile relies on the engine to provide motion, the body depends on the muscular system to perform both voluntary and involuntary movements. Walking, breathing, and the digestion of food are but a few examples of body functions that require the healthy performance of the muscular system.

Although this system has several functions, the primary purpose is to provide movement or power. Muscles produce power by contracting. The ability of a large muscle or muscle group to contract depends on the ability of microscopic muscle fibers to contract within the larger muscle. An understanding of these microscopic muscle fibers will assist you as you progress in your study to the larger muscles and muscle groups.

Muscle contractions may be one of several types: isotonic, isometric, twitch, or tetanic. When skeletal or voluntary muscles contract, they provide us with a variety of motions. Flexion, extension, abduction, adduction, and rotation are examples of these movements that provide us with both strength and agility.

Muscles are also used to keep the body healthy and in good condition. Scientific evidence keeps pointing to the fact that the proper use and exercise of muscles may prolong longevity. An understanding of the structure and function of the muscular system may, therefore, add quality and quantity to our lives.

TOPICS FOR REVIEW

Before progressing to Chapter 9, you should familiarize yourself with the structure and function of the three major types of muscle tissue. Your review should include the microscopic structure of skeletal muscle tissue, how a muscle is stimulated, the major types of skeletal muscle contractions, and the skeletal muscle groups. Your study should conclude with an understanding of the types of movements produced by skeletal muscle contractions and the major muscular disorders.

MUSCLE TISSUE

Match each descriptive word or phrase to its related muscle type and write the corresponding letter(s) in the answer blank.

A. Skeletal muscle   B. Cardiac muscle   C. Smooth muscle

_____ 1.   Striated

_____ 2.   Cells branch frequently

_____ 3.   Moves food into the stomach

_____ 4.   Nonstriated

_____ 5.   Voluntary

_____ 6.   Keeps blood circulating through its vessels

_____ 7.   Involuntary

_____ 8.   Attaches to bone

_____ 9.   Hollow internal organs

_____ 10.   Visceral muscle

▶ *If you had difficulty with this section, review pages 207-208.*

STRUCTURE OF SKELETAL MUSCLES

Match each term on the left with its corresponding description on the right.

_____ 11. Origin   A. The muscle unit excluding the ends
_____ 12. Insertion   B. Attachment to the more movable bone
_____ 13. Body   C. Fluid-filled sacs
_____ 14. Tendons   D. Attachment to more stationary bone
_____ 15. Bursae   E. Anchor muscles to bones

MICROSCOPIC STRUCTURE

_____ 16. Muscle fibers   A. Protein that forms thick myofilaments
_____ 17. Actin   B. Basic functional unit of skeletal muscle
_____ 18. Sarcomere   C. Protein that forms thin myofilaments
_____ 19. Myosin   D. Microscopic threadlike structures found in skeletal muscle fibers
_____ 20. Myofilaments   E. Elongated contractile cells of muscle tissue

▶ *If you had difficulty with this section, review pages 208-211.*

FUNCTIONS OF SKELETAL MUSCLE

Fill in the blanks.

21. Muscles move bones by _____ on them.

22. As a rule, only the _____ bone moves.

23. The _____ bone moves toward the _____ bone.

24. Of all the muscles contracting simultaneously, the one mainly responsible for producing a particular movement is called the _____ _____ for that movement.

25. As prime movers contract, other muscles called _____ relax.

26. The biceps brachii is the prime mover during flexing, and the brachialis is its helper or _____ muscle.

27. We are able to maintain our body position because of a specialized type of skeletal muscle contraction called _____ _____.

28. _____ _____ maintains body posture by counteracting the pull of gravity.

29. A decrease in temperature, a condition known as _____, will drastically affect cellular activity and normal body function.

30. Energy required to produce a muscle contraction is obtained from _____.

▷ *If you had difficulty with this section, review page 211.*

FATIGUE
ROLE OF OTHER BODY SYSTEMS
MOTOR UNIT
MUSCLE STIMULUS

If the statement is true, write "T" in the answer blank. If the statement is false, correct the statement by circling the incorrect term and writing the correct term in the answer blank.

_____ 31. The point of contact between the nerve ending and the muscle fiber is called a *motor neuron*.

_____ 32. A motor neuron together with the cells it innervates is called a *motor unit*.

_____ 33. If muscle cells are stimulated repeatedly without adequate periods of rest, the strength of the muscle contraction will decrease resulting in fatigue.

_____ 34. The depletion of oxygen in muscle cells during vigorous and prolonged exercise is known as *fatigue*.

_____ 35. An adequate stimulus will contract a muscle cell completely because of the "must" theory.

_____ 36. When oxygen supplies run low, muscle cells produce ATP and other waste products during contraction.

_____ 37. In a laboratory setting, a single muscle fiber can be isolated and subjected to stimuli of varying intensities so that it can be studied.

_____ 38. The minimal level of stimulation required to cause a fiber to contract is called the _threshold stimulus_.

_____ 39. Smooth muscles bring about movements by pulling on bones across movable joints.

_____ 40. A nervous system disorder that shuts off impulses to certain skeletal muscles may result in paralysis.

TYPES OF SKELETAL MUSCLE CONTRACTION

Circle the correct answer.

41. When a muscle contracts and no movement results, the contraction is:
    A. Isometric
    B. Isotonic
    C. Twitch
    D. Tetanic

42. Walking is an example of which type of contraction?
    A. Isometric
    B. Isotonic
    C. Twitch
    D. Tetanic

43. Pushing against a wall is an example of which type of contraction?
    A. Isotonic
    B. Isometric
    C. Twitch
    D. Tetanic

44. Endurance training is also known as:
    A. Isometrics
    B. Hypertrophy
    C. Aerobic training
    D. Strength training

45. Benefits of regular exercise include all of the following _except_:
    A. Improved lung functioning
    B. More efficient heart
    C. Less fatigue
    D. Atrophy

46. Twitch contractions easily can be seen:
    A. In isolated muscles prepared for research
    B. In a great deal of normal muscle activity
    C. During resting periods
    D. None of the above

47. Individual contractions "melt" together to produce a sustained contraction or:
    A. Twitch
    B. Tetanus
    C. Isotonic response
    D. Isometric response

48. In most cases, isotonic contraction of muscle produces movement at a/an:
    A. Insertion
    B. Beginning
    C. Joint
    D. Bursa

49. Prolonged inactivity causes muscles to shrink in mass, a condition called:
    A. Hypertrophy
    B. Disuse atrophy
    C. Paralysis
    D. Muscle fatigue

50. Muscle hypertrophy can be best enhanced by a program of:
    A. Isotonic exercise
    B. Better posture
    C. High-protein diet
    D. Strength training

▶ _If you have had difficulty with this section, review pages 211-216._

SKELETAL MUSCLE GROUPS

Match the function(s) to the muscles listed below and write the corresponding letter(s) in the answer blank.

A. Flexor   C. Abductor   E. Rotator
B. Extensor   D. Adductor   F. Dorsiflexor or plantar flexor

_____ 51. Deltoid

_____ 52. Tibialis anterior

_____ 53. Gastrocnemius

_____ 54. Biceps brachii

_____ 55. Gluteus medius

_____ 56. Soleus

_____ 57. Iliopsoas

_____ 58. Pectoralis major

_____ 59. Gluteus maximus

_____ 60. Triceps brachii

_____ 61. Sternocleidomastoid

_____ 62. Trapezius

_____ 63. Gracilis

▶ *If you had difficulty with this section, review pages 216-221 and 223.*

MOVEMENTS PRODUCED BY SKELETAL MUSCLE CONTRACTIONS

Circle the correct answer.

64. A movement that makes the angle between two bones smaller is:
   A. Flexion
   B. Extension
   C. Abduction
   D. Adduction

65. Moving a part toward the midline is:
   A. Flexion
   B. Extension
   C. Abduction
   D. Adduction

66. Moving a part away from the midline is:
   A. Flexion
   B. Extension
   C. Abduction
   D. Adduction

67. When you move your head from side to side as in shaking your head "no," you are _____ a muscle group.
   A. Rotating
   B. Pronating
   C. Supinating
   D. Abducting

68. _____ occurs when you turn the palm of your hand from an anterior to posterior position.
   A. Dorsiflexion
   B. Plantar flexion
   C. Supination
   D. Pronation

69. *Dorsiflexion* refers to:
   A. Hand movements
   B. Eye movements
   C. Foot movements
   D. Head movements

▶ *If you had difficulty with this section, review pages 221-223.*

MAJOR MUSCULAR DISORDERS

Circle the correct answer.

70. Muscle strains are characterized by (*myalgia* or *fibromyositis*).

71. Crush injuries can cause (*hemoglobin* or *myoglobin*) to accumulate in the blood and result in kidney failure.

72. A viral infection of the nerves that controls skeletal muscle movement is known as (*poliomyelitis* or *muscular dystrophy*).

73. (*Muscular dystrophy* or *Myasthenia gravis*) is a group of genetic diseases characterized by atrophy of skeletal muscle tissues.

74. (*Muscular dystrophy* or *Myasthenia gravis*) is an autoimmune disease in which the immune system attacks muscle cells at the neuromuscular junction.

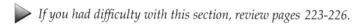 *If you had difficulty with this section, review pages 223-226.*

APPLYING WHAT YOU KNOW

75. Casey noticed pain whenever she reached for anything in her cupboards. Her doctor told her that the small fluid-filled sacs in her shoulder were inflamed. What condition did Casey have?

76. The nurse was preparing an injection for Mrs. Tatakis. The amount to be given was 2 mL. What area of the body will the nurse most likely select for administering this injection?

77. Chris was playing football and pulled a band of fibrous connective tissue that attached a muscle to a bone. What is the common term for this tissue?

78.   Word Find

Find and circle 25 muscle terms. Words may be spelled top to bottom, bottom to top, right to left, left to right, or diagonally.

```
G  A  S  T  R  O  C  N  E  M  I  U  S  D  U
M  S  G  I  O  N  O  I  S  N  E  T  X  E  U
U  R  N  N  T  O  M  S  R  B  S  F  D  T  T
S  U  I  S  C  I  B  O  N  T  P  N  E  A  R
C  B  R  E  U  X  V  T  O  O  E  C  L  I  A
L  Q  T  R  D  E  C  O  D  A  C  M  T  R  P
E  T  S  T  B  L  M  N  N  V  I  E  O  T  E
X  F  M  I  A  F  Y  I  E  Y  B  N  I  S  Z
S  I  A  O  V  I  E  C  T  L  S  S  D  I  I
S  Y  H  N  S  S  R  O  T  A  T  O  R  G  U
U  A  M  G  A  R  H  P  A  I  D  J  N  R  S
E  H  A  T  R  O  P  H  Y  L  N  J  T  E  B
L  N  O  H  T  D  E  U  G  I  T  A  F  N  T
O  R  I  G  I  N  O  S  N  V  S  B  Z  Y  L
S  B  V  T  O  J  C  T  R  I  C  E  P  S  S
```

Abductor	Flexion	Soleus
Atrophy	Gastrocnemius	Striated
Biceps	Hamstrings	Synergist
Bursa	Insertion	Tendon
Deltoid	Isometric	Tenosynovitis
Diaphragm	Isotonic	Trapezius
Dorsiflexion	Muscle	Triceps
Extension	Origin	
Fatigue	Rotator	

DID YOU KNOW?

If all of your muscles pulled in one direction, you would have the power to move 25 tons.

THE MUSCULAR SYSTEM

Fill in the crossword puzzle.

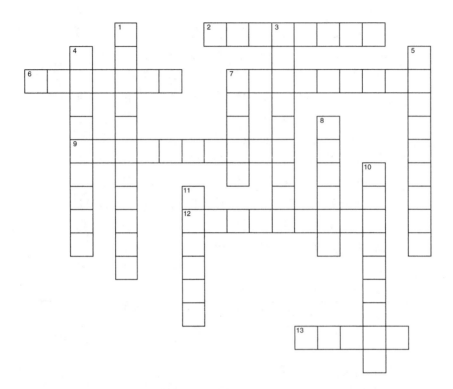

ACROSS

2. Shaking your head "no"
6. Muscle shrinkage
7. Toward the body's midline
9. Produces movement opposite to prime movers
12. Movement that makes joint angles larger
13. Small fluid-filled sac between tendons and bones

DOWN

1. Increase in size
3. Away from the body's midline
4. Turning your palm from an anterior to posterior position
5. Attachment to the more movable bone
7. Protein which composes myofilaments
8. Attachment to the more stationary bone
10. Assists prime movers with movement
11. Anchors muscles to bones

CHECK YOUR KNOWLEDGE

Multiple Choice

Circle the correct answer.

1. Which of the following statements about a motor unit is true?
   A. It consists of a muscle cell group and a motor neuron.
   B. The point of contact between the nerve ending and the muscle fiber is called the *neuromuscular junction.*
   C. Chemicals generate events within the muscle cell that result in contraction of the muscle cell.
   D. All of the above are true.

2. What is movement of a part away from the midline of the body called?
   A. Abduction
   B. Adduction
   C. Pronation
   D. Plantar flexion

3. According to the sliding filament theory of muscle contraction:
   A. Muscle fibers contain thin myofilaments made of a protein called *myosin.*
   B. Muscle fibers contain thick myofilaments made up of a protein called *actin.*
   C. Thin and thick myofilaments move toward each other to cause muscle contraction.
   D. All of the above are true.

4. Which of the following statements is true of the hamstring group of muscles?
   A. It includes the rectus femoris.
   B. It flexes the knee.
   C. It originates on the pubis.
   D. All of the above are true.

5. What happens if a given muscle cell is stimulated by a threshold stimulus?
   A. It shows an "all or none" response.
   B. It shows a tetanus response.
   C. It shows a subminimal response.
   D. None of the above is true.

6. Which of the following statements about oxygen debt is true?
   A. It is caused when excess oxygen is present in the environment.
   B. It causes lactic acid buildup and soreness in muscles.
   C. It can be replaced by slow, shallow breathing.
   D. All of the above are true.

7. What is a quick, jerky response of a given muscle to a single stimulus called?
   A. Isometric
   B. Lockjaw
   C. Tetanus
   D. Twitch

8. Which of the following statements about muscle atrophy is true?
   A. It decreases the size of a muscle.
   B. It increases the size of a muscle.
   C. Has no effect on muscle size.
   D. None of the above is true.

9. Which of the following occurs during isometric exercises?
   A. Muscle length remains the same.
   B. Muscle tension remains the same.
   C. Muscle length shortens.
   D. None of the above occurs.

10. Which of the following statements about skeletal muscle contraction is true?
    A. Its attachment to the more stationary bone is called its *origin.*
    B. Its attachment to the more moveable bone is called its *insertion.*
    C. Both A and B are true.
    D. None of the above is true.

True/False

If the statement is true, write "T" on the answer blank. If the statement is false, correct the statement by circling the incorrect term and writing the correct term in the answer blank.

_____ 11. When a part is moved toward the midline, it is called *adduction*.

_____ 12. In most cases, isotonic contraction of a muscle produces movement at a joint.

_____ 13. Dorsiflexion occurs when you turn the palm of your hand from an anterior to a posterior position.

_____ 14. Exercise may cause an increase in muscle size called *atrophy*.

_____ 15. Isotonic contraction is an example of a contraction used while walking.

_____ 16. If a muscle is overworked without sufficient rest, the result will be a decrease in muscle strength and fatigue.

_____ 17. A bone of insertion moves toward the bone of origin.

_____ 18. A condition in which the body temperature is drastically low is referred to as *hyperthermia*.

_____ 19. Tetanic contraction is caused by a series of rapid stimuli.

_____ 20. When the angle between two bones becomes smaller, it is called *extension*.

MUSCLES—ANTERIOR VIEW

1. _____

2. _____

3. _____

4. _____

5. _____

6. _____

7. _____

8. _____

9. _____

10. _____

11. _____

12. _____

13. _____

14. _____

15. _____

16. _____

17. _____

18. _____

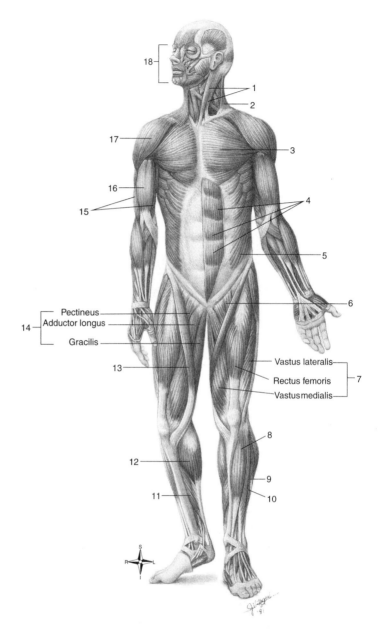

MUSCLES—POSTERIOR VIEW

1. _____

2. _____

3. _____

4. _____

5. _____

6. _____

7. _____

8. _____

9. _____

10. _____

11. _____

12. _____

13. _____

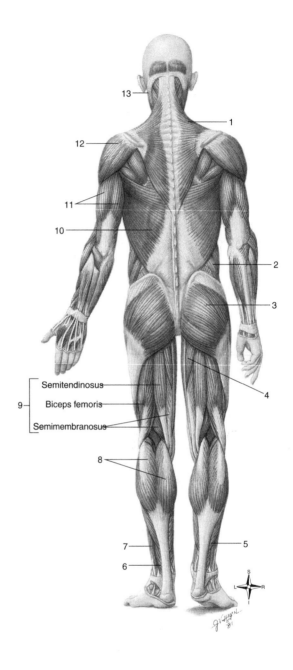

The Nervous System

T he nervous system organizes and coordinates the millions of impulses received each day to make communication with and enjoyment of our environment possible. The functioning unit of the nervous system is the neuron. Three types of neurons exist—sensory, motor, and interneurons—which are classified according to the direction in which they transmit impulses. Nerve impulses travel over routes made up of neurons and provide the rapid communication necessary for maintaining life. The central nervous system is made up of the spinal cord and brain. The spinal cord provides access to and from the brain by means of ascending and descending tracts. In addition, the spinal cord functions as the primary reflex center of the body. The brain consists of the brainstem, cerebellum, diencephalon, and cerebrum. These areas provide the extraordinary network necessary to receive, interpret, and respond to the simplest or most complex impulses.

While you concentrate on this chapter, your body is performing a multitude of functions. Fortunately for us, the beating of the heart, the digestion of food, breathing, and most of our other day-to-day processes do not require our supervision or thought. They function automatically, and the division of the nervous system that regulates these functions is known as the *autonomic nervous system*. The autonomic nervous system consists of two divisions called the *sympathetic system* and the *parasympathetic system*. The sympathetic system functions as an emergency system and prepares us for "fight or flight." The parasympathetic system dominates control of many visceral effectors under normal everyday conditions. Together, these two divisions regulate the body's automatic functions in an effort to assist with the maintenance of homeostasis. Your understanding of this chapter will help you comprehend the complex functions of the nervous system and the "automatic pilot" of your body—the autonomic system.

TOPICS FOR REVIEW

Before progressing to Chapter 10, you should review the organs and divisions of the nervous system, the structure and function of the major types of cells in this system, the structure and function of a reflex arc, and the transmission of nerve impulses. Your study should include the anatomy and physiology of the brain and spinal cord and the nerves that extend from these two areas. Finally, an understanding of the autonomic nervous system, the specific functions of the subdivisions of this system, and the major disorders of the nervous system are necessary to complete the review of this chapter.

ORGANS AND DIVISIONS OF THE NERVOUS SYSTEM
CELLS OF THE NERVOUS SYSTEM
NERVES

Match each term on the left with the most appropriate description on the right.

Group A

_____ 1. Sense organ
_____ 2. Central nervous system
_____ 3. Peripheral nervous system
_____ 4. Autonomic nervous system

A. Subdivision of peripheral nervous system
B. Ear
C. Brain and spinal cord
D. Nerves that extend to the outlying parts of the body

Group B

_____ 5. Dendrite
_____ 6. Schwann cell
_____ 7. Motor neuron
_____ 8. Nodes of Ranvier
_____ 9. Fascicles
_____ 10. Epineurium

A. Indentations between adjacent Schwann cells
B. Branching projection of neuron
C. Also known as *efferent*
D. Forms myelin outside the CNS
E. Tough sheath that covers the whole nerve
F. Groups of wrapped axons

CELLS OF NERVOUS SYSTEM
NERVES

Match each of the following words or phrases to its corresponding nervous system structure. Write the correct letter in the answer blank.

A. Neurons   B. Neuroglia

_____ 11. Axon

_____ 12. Supporting cells

_____ 13. Astrocytes

_____ 14. Sensory

_____ 15. Conduct impulses

_____ 16. Form the myelin sheath around central nerve fibers

_____ 17. Phagocytosis

_____ 18. Efferent

_____ 19. Multiple sclerosis

_____ 20. Neurilemma

▶ *If you had difficulty with this section, review pages 235-240.*

REFLEX ARCS

Fill in the blanks.

21. The simplest kind of reflex arc is a _____
    _____ _____.

22. Three-neuron arcs consist of all three kinds of neurons, _____,
    _____, and _____
    _____.

23. Impulse conduction in a reflex arc normally starts in _____.

24. A _____ is the microscopic space that separates the axon of one neuron
    from the dendrites of another neuron.

25. A _____ is the response to impulse conduction over reflex arcs.

26. Contraction of a muscle that causes it to pull away from an irritating stimulus is known as the
    _____ _____.

27. A _____ is a group of nerve-cell bodies located in the peripheral ner-
    vous system.

28. All _____ lie entirely within the gray matter of the central nervous sys-
    tem.

29. In a patellar reflex, the nerve impulses that reach the quadriceps muscle (the effector) result in the classic
    _____ _____ response.

30. _____ _____ forms the H-shaped
    inner core of the spinal cord.

▷ *If you had difficulty with this section, review pages 240-242.*

NERVE IMPULSES
THE SYNAPSE

Circle the correct answer.

31. Nerve impulses (*do* or *do not*) continually race along every nerve cell's surface.

32. When a stimulus acts on a neuron, it (*increases* or *decreases*) the permeability of the stimulated point of its
    membrane to sodium ions.

33. An inward movement of positive ions leaves a/an (*lack* or *excess*) of negative ions outside.

34. The plasma membrane of the (*presynaptic* or *postsynaptic*) neuron makes up a portion of the synapse.

35. A synaptic knob is a tiny bulge at the end of the (*presynaptic* or *postsynaptic*) neuron's axon.

36. Acetylcholine is an example of a (*neurotransmitter* or *protein molecule receptor*).

37. Neurotransmitters are chemicals that allow neurons to (*communicate* or *reproduce*) with one another.

38. Neurotransmitters are distributed (*randomly* or *specifically*) into groups of neurons.

39. Catecholamines may play a role in (*sleep* or *reproduction*).

40. Endorphins and enkephalins are neurotransmitters that inhibit conduction of (*fear* or *pain*) impulses.

▷ *If you had difficulty with this section, review pages 242-246.*

CENTRAL NERVOUS SYSTEM
DIVISIONS OF THE BRAIN

Circle the correct answer.

41. The portion of the brainstem that joins the spinal cord to the brain is the:
    A. Pons
    B. Cerebellum
    C. Diencephalon
    D. Hypothalamus
    E. Medulla

42. Which one of the following is *not* a function of the brainstem?
    A. Conducts sensory impulses from the spinal cord to the higher centers of the brain.
    B. Conducts motor impulses from the cerebrum to the spinal cord.
    C. Controls heartbeat, respiration, and blood vessel diameter.
    D. Contains centers for speech and memory.

43. Which one of the following is *not* part of the diencephalon?
    A. Cerebrum
    B. Thalamus
    C. Pituitary gland
    D. Third ventricle gray matter

44. ADH is produced by the:
    A. Pituitary gland
    B. Medulla
    C. Mammillary bodies
    D. Third ventricle
    E. Hypothalamus

45. Which one of the following is *not* a function of the hypothalamus?
    A. It helps control the heart rate.
    B. It helps control the constriction and dilation of blood vessels.
    C. It helps control the contraction of the stomach and intestines.
    D. It produces hormones that control the release of certain anterior pituitary hormones.
    E. All of the above are functions of the hypothalamus.

46. Which one of the following parts of the brain helps in the association of sensations with emotions, as well as aiding in the arousal or alerting mechanism?
    A. Pons
    B. Hypothalamus
    C. Cerebellum
    D. Thalamus
    E. None of the above is correct

47. Which of the following is *not* true of the cerebrum?
    A. Its lobes correspond to the bones that lie over them.
    B. Its grooves are called *gyri*.
    C. Most of its gray matter lies on the surface of the cerebrum.
    D. Its outer region is called the *cerebral cortex*.
    E. Its two hemispheres are connected by a structure called the *corpus callosum*.

48. Which one of the following is *not* a function of the cerebrum?
    A. Willed movement
    B. Consciousness
    C. Memory
    D. Conscious awareness of sensations
    E. All of the above are functions of the cerebrum

49. The area of the cerebrum responsible for the perception of sound lies in the _____ lobe.
    A. Frontal
    B. Temporal
    C. Occipital
    D. Parietal

50. Visual perception is located in the _____ lobe.
    A. Frontal
    B. Temporal
    C. Parietal
    D. Occipital
    E. None of the above is correct

51. Which one of the following is *not* a function of the cerebellum?
    A. Maintains equilibrium
    B. Helps produce smooth, coordinated movements
    C. Helps maintain normal postures
    D. Associates sensations with emotions

52. Within the interior of the cerebrum are a few islands of gray matter known as:
    A. Fissures
    B. Basal ganglia
    C. Gyri
    D. Myelin

53. A cerebrovascular accident is commonly referred to as (a):
    A. Stroke
    B. Parkinson disease
    C. Tumor
    D. Multiple sclerosis

54. Parkinson disease is a disease of the:
    A. Myelin
    B. Axons
    C. Neuroglia
    D. Cerebral nuclei

55. The largest section of the brain is the:
    A. Cerebellum
    B. Pons
    C. Cerebrum
    D. Midbrain

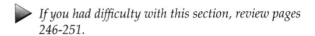 *If you had difficulty with this section, review pages 246-251.*

BRAIN STUDIES

BRAIN DISORDERS

Match each numbered description to the most appropriate term and write the corresponding letter in the answer blank.

A. SPECT
B. MRI
C. CT
D. Hemiplegia
E. Cerebral palsy

F. EEG
G. Huntington disease
H. CVA
I. Dementia
J. PET

_____ 56. Stroke

_____ 57. Paralysis of one side of the body

_____ 58. A crippling disease that involves permanent, nonprogressive damage to motor control areas of the brain

_____ 59. An imaging technique for the brain that involves scanning the head with a revolving x-ray generator

_____ 60. A scanning method that determines the functional characteristics of the brain by introducing a radioactive substance into the blood supply of the brain

_____ 61. Used to visualize blood flow in the brain

_____ 62. A scanning method that uses a magnetic field to induce brain tissues to emit radio waves

_____ 63. Measurement of electrical activity of the brain

_____ 64. Characteristic of Alzheimer disease

_____ 65. Inherited disease characterized by chorea

If you had difficulty with this section, review pages 251-255.

SPINAL CORD

If the statement is true, write "T" in the answer blank. If the statement is false, correct the statement by circling the incorrect term and writing the correct term in the answer blank.

_____ 66. The spinal cord is approximately 24 to 25 inches long.

_____ 67. The spinal cord ends at the bottom of the sacrum.

_____ 68. The extension of the meninges beyond the cord is convenient for performing CAT scans without danger of injuring the spinal cord.

_____ 69. Bundles of myelinated nerve fibers—dendrites—make up the white outer columns of the spinal cord.

_____ 70. Ascending tracts conduct impulses up the cord to the brain and descending tracts conduct impulses down the cord from the brain.

_____ 71. Tracts are functional organizations in that all of the axons that compose a tract serve several functions.

_____ 72. A loss of sensation caused by a spinal cord injury is called *paralysis*.

▷ *If you had difficulty with this section, review pages 255-257.*

COVERINGS AND FLUID SPACES OF THE BRAIN AND SPINAL CORD

Circle the word in each word group that does not belong.

73. Meninges   Pia mater   Ventricles   Dura mater
74. Arachnoid   Middle layer   CSF   Cobweb-like
75. CSF   Ventricles   Subarachnoid space   Pia mater
76. Tough   Outer layer   Dura mater   Choroid plexus
77. Brain tumor   Subarachnoid space   CSF   Fourth lumbar vertebra

CRANIAL NERVES

78. Fill in the missing areas on the chart below.

NERVE		CONDUCT IMPULSES	FUNCTION
I		From nose to brain	Sense of smell
II	Optic	From eye to brain	
III	Oculomotor		Eye movements
IV		From brain to external eye muscles	Eye movements
V	Trigeminal	From skin and mucous membrane of head and from teeth to brain; also from brain to chewing muscles	

VI	Abducens		Eye movements
VII	Facial	From taste buds of tongue to brain; from brain to face muscles	
VIII		From ear to brain	Hearing; sense of balance
IX	Glossopharyngeal		Sensations of throat, taste, swallowing movements, secretion of saliva
X		From throat, larynx, and organs in thoracic and abdominal cavities to brain; also from brain to muscles of throat and abdominal cavities	Sensations of throat, larynx, and of thoracic and abdominal organs; swallowing, voice production, slowing of heartbeat, acceleration of peristalsis (gut movements)
XI	Accessory	From brain to certain shoulder and neck muscles	
XII		From brain to muscles of tongue	Tongue movements

 If you had difficulty with this section, review pages 257-260 and Table 9-23.

CRANIAL NERVES

SPINAL NERVES

Match each of the numbered words with cranial or spinal nerves as appropriate and write the corresponding letter in the answer blank.

A. Cranial nerves   B.   Spinal nerves

_____ 79.   12 pairs

_____ 80.   Dermatome

_____ 81.   Vagus

_____ 82.   Shingles

_____ 83.   31 pairs

_____ 84.   Optic

_____ 85.   C1

_____ 86.   Plexus

 If you had difficulty with this section, review pages 260-264.

AUTONOMIC NERVOUS SYSTEM

Match each term on the left with the appropriate description on the right.

_____ 87.   Autonomic nervous system

_____ 88.   Autonomic neurons

_____ 89.   Preganglionic neurons

_____ 90.   Visceral effectors

_____ 91.   Sympathetic nervous system

_____ 92.   Somatic nervous system

A.   Divisions of ANS

B.   Tissues to which autonomic neurons conduct impulses

C.   Voluntary actions

D.   Regulates body's involuntary functions

E.   Motor neurons that make up the ANS

F.   Conduct impulses between the spinal cord and a ganglion

SYMPATHETIC NERVOUS SYSTEM

PARASYMPATHETIC NERVOUS SYSTEM

Circle the correct answer.

93. Dendrites and cell bodies of sympathetic pre-ganglionic neurons are located in the:
    A.   Brainstem and sacral portion of the spinal cord
    B.   Sympathetic ganglia
    C.   Gray matter of the thoracic and upper lumbar segments of the spinal cord
    D.   Ganglia close to effectors

94. Which of the following is *not* correct?
    A.   Sympathetic preganglionic neurons have their cell bodies located in the lateral gray column of certain parts of the spinal cord.
    B.   Sympathetic preganglionic axons pass along the dorsal root of certain spinal nerves.
    C.   There are synapses within sympathetic ganglia.
    D.   Sympathetic responses are usually widespread, involving many organs.

95. Another name for the parasympathetic nervous system is:
    A.   Thoracolumbar
    B.   Craniosacral
    C.   Visceral
    D.   ANS
    E.   Cholinergic

96. Which statement is *not* correct?
    A.   Sympathetic postganglionic neurons have their dendrites and cell bodies in sympathetic ganglia or collateral ganglia.
    B.   Sympathetic ganglions are located in front of and at each side of the spinal column.
    C.   Separate autonomic nerves distribute many sympathetic postganglionic axons to various internal organs.
    D.   Very few sympathetic preganglionic axons synapse with postganglionic neurons.

97. Sympathetic stimulation usually results in a/an:
    A.   Response by numerous organs
    B.   Response by only one organ
    C.   Increase in peristalsis
    D.   Constriction of pupils

98. Parasympathetic stimulation frequently results in a/an:
    A.   Response by only one organ
    B.   Response by numerous organs
    C.   Fight-or-flight syndrome
    D.   Increase in heartbeat

Match each numbered description to its related nervous control system and write the corresponding letter in answer blanks.

A. Sympathetic control   B. Parasympathetic control

_____ 99.   Constricts pupils

_____ 100. "Goose pimples"

_____ 101. Increases sweat secretion

_____ 102. Increases secretion of digestive juices

_____ 103. Constricts blood vessels

_____ 104. Slows heartbeat

_____ 105. Relaxes bladder

_____ 106. Increases epinephrine secretion

_____ 107. Increases peristalsis

_____ 108. Stimulates lens for near vision

▶ *If you had difficulty with this section, review pages 264-268.*

AUTONOMIC NEUROTRANSMITTERS
AUTONOMIC NERVOUS SYSTEM AS A WHOLE

Fill in the blanks.

109. Sympathetic preganglionic axons release the neurotransmitter _____.

110. Axons that release norepinephrine are classified as _____
      _____.

111. Axons that release acetylcholine are classified as _____
      _____.

112. The function of the autonomic nervous system is to regulate the body's involuntary functions in ways
      that maintain or restore _____.

113. Your _____ _____ is determined
      by the combined forces of the sympathetic and parasympathetic nervous systems.

114. According to some physiologists, meditation leads to _____ sympa-
      thetic activity and changes opposite to those of the fight-or-flight response.

115. _____ is a malignant tumor of the sympathetic nervous system.

▶ *If you had difficulty with this section, review pages 268-270.*

UNSCRAMBLE THE WORDS

116. **R O N N E S U**

[ ][ ][ ][ ][ ][ ][(O)]

117. **A P S Y E N S**

[ ][(O)][ ][(O) (O)][ ][ ]

118. **C I A T U N O M O**

[ ][ ][(O)][ ][ ][(O) (O)][ ]

119. **S H T O M O   U L M S E C**

[ ][ ][ ][(O) (O)][ ] [ ][ ][ ][(O)][(O)]

Take the circled letters, unscramble them, and fill in the solution.

What the man hoped the IRS agent would be during his audit.

120. [ ][ ][ ][ ][ ][ ][ ][ ][ ][ ][ ][ ]

APPLYING WHAT YOU KNOW

121. Mr. Hemstreet suffered a cerebrovascular accident, and it was determined that the resulting damage affected the left side of his cerebrum. On which side of his body will he most likely notice any paralysis?

122. Baby Dania was born with an excessive accumulation of cerebrospinal fluid in the ventricles. A catheter was placed in the ventricle and the fluid was drained by means of a shunt into the circulatory bloodstream. What condition does this medical history describe?

123. Mrs. Muhlenkamp looked out her window to see a man trapped under the wheel of a car. Although slightly built, Mrs. Muhlenkamp rushed to the car, lifted it, and saved the man. What division of the autonomic nervous system made this seemingly impossible task possible?

124. Lynn's heart raced and her palms became clammy as she watched the monster at the local theater. When the movie was over, however, she told her friends that she was not afraid at all. She appeared to be as calm as before the movie. What division of the autonomic nervous system made this possible?

125. Bill is scheduled to meet with his boss for his annual evaluation. He is planning to ask for a raise and hopes the evaluation will be good. Which subdivision of the autonomic nervous system will be active during this conference? Should he have a large meal before his appointment? Support your answer with facts from the chapter.

126. Word Find

Find and circle 14 terms presented in this chapter. Words may be spelled top to bottom, bottom to top, right to left, left to right, or diagonally.

```
M  C  C  D  Q  S  Y  N  A  P  S  E  Q  G  O
E  N  A  Q  D  W  H  N  W  E  J  N  A  L  W
S  R  O  T  P  E  C  E  R  Y  Z  N  I  S  M
I  D  S  X  E  K  N  O  K  X  G  G  C  Y  Y
J  O  T  R  A  C  T  D  F  L  O  N  E  N  A
R  P  W  E  K  O  H  X  I  D  A  L  H  A  M
F  A  L  O  N  A  Y  O  E  I  I  I  X  P  C
C  M  Z  I  F  D  N  N  L  N  G  Z  U  T  Z
S  I  N  V  C  G  D  G  Z  A  N  A  K  I  P
G  N  A  T  Z  R  O  W  V  A  M  Y  T  C  O
K  E  N  D  O  R  P  H  I  N  S  I  L  C  X
C  P  Q  G  C  J  X  F  J  D  Q  S  N  L  F
X  U  L  I  H  I  G  Q  A  N  S  W  O  E  U
A  I  M  H  Q  E  X  K  D  B  W  Y  T  F  S
A  A  D  A  X  O  C  K  G  B  F  H  B  T  K
```

Axon	Glia	Serotonin
Catecholamines	Microglia	Synapse
Dopamine	Myelin	Synaptic cleft
Endorphins	Oligodendroglia	Tract
Ganglion	Receptors	

DID YOU KNOW?

Although all pain is felt and interpreted in the brain, the brain itself has no pain sensation—even when cut!

THE NERVOUS SYSTEM

Fill in the crossword puzzle.

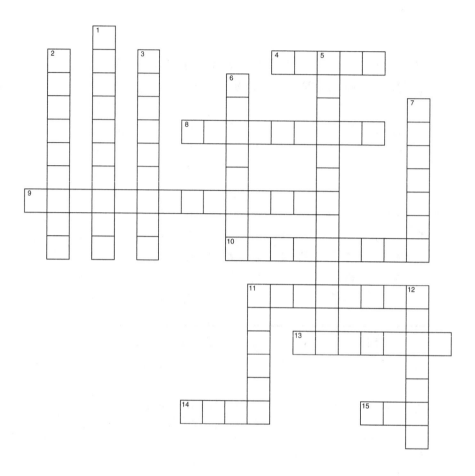

ACROSS

4. Bundle of axons located within the CNS
8. Transmits impulses toward the cell body
9. Neurons that conduct impulses from a ganglion
10. Astrocytes
11. Pia mater
13. Nerve cells
14. Transmits impulses away from the cell body
15. Peripheral nervous system (abbreviation)

DOWN

1. Neuroglia
2. Peripheral beginning of a sensory neuron's dendrite
3. Two-neuron arc (two words)
5. Neurotransmitter
6. Cluster of nerve cell bodies outside the central nervous system
7. Area of brain stem

11. Fatty substance found around some nerve fibers
12. Where impulses are transmitted from one neuron to another

CHECK YOUR KNOWLEDGE

Multiple Choice

Circle the correct answer.

1. What are the neurons called that pick up sensations from receptors and carry them into the brain or spinal cord?
   A. Motor neurons
   B. Central neurons
   C. Interneurons
   D. Sensory neurons

2. What are the brain cavities called that are filled with cerebrospinal fluid?
   A. Hydrocephalics
   B. Ventricles
   C. Mater
   D. Meninges

3. What is the innermost layer of connective tissue that surrounds the brain and spinal cord?
   A. Pia mater
   B. Dura mater
   C. Arachnoid mater
   D. Pons mater

4. A nurse is caring for a patient with a tumor of the cerebellum. In view of the functions of this part of the brain, which of the following symptoms should the nurse expect to observe?
   A. Irregular heartbeat and increased blood pressure
   B. Inability to coordinate body movements
   C. Loss of speech
   D. Inability to control emotions

5. What occurs as a result of stimulation of the sympathetic nervous system?
   A. Accelerated heart rate
   B. Constriction of blood vessels in skeletal muscles
   C. Increased peristalsis
   D. All of the above

6. The autonomic neurotransmitter called *acetylcholine* is released by the:
   A. Sympathetic preganglionic axon
   B. Parasympathetic preganglionic axon
   C. Parasympathetic postganglionic axon
   D. All of the above

7. Which of the following statements about Schwann cells is true?
   A. They are found in the PNS.
   B. They produce myelin.
   C. They are separated by nodes of Ranvier.
   D. All of the above are true.

8. What are areas of the neuron called that secrete neurotransmitters?
   A. Synapses
   B. Synaptic clefts
   C. Synaptic knobs
   D. Gliomas

9. Which of the following statements about the neural tissues called *tracts* is true?
   A. They are located outside of the central nervous system.
   B. They appear gray.
   C. When carrying messages upward they are called *ascending*, and when carrying messages downward they are called *descending*.
   D. All of the above are true.

10. Which of the following statements about the autonomic division of the nervous system is true?
    A. It is composed of two divisions: the sympathetic and parasympathetic.
    B. Autonomic neurotransmitters assist the system in its effort to elicit responses.
    C. The system regulates the body's involuntary functions.
    D. All of the above are true.

Matching

Match each term in column A with its corresponding description in column B. (Only one answer is correct for each.)

Column A

_____ 11. Tract

_____ 12. Axon

_____ 13. Brain stem

_____ 14. Neurotransmitter

_____ 15. Central neuron

_____ 16. Skin map

_____ 17. Brain tumor

_____ 18. Diencephalon

_____ 19. Vagus

_____ 20. Limbic system

Column B

A.   Transmits away from the cell body

B.   Interneuron

C.   White matter

D.   Cranial nerve

E.   Thalamus

F.   Glioma

G.   Emotional brain

H.   Acetylcholine

I.   Dermatome

J.   Medulla oblongata

NEURON

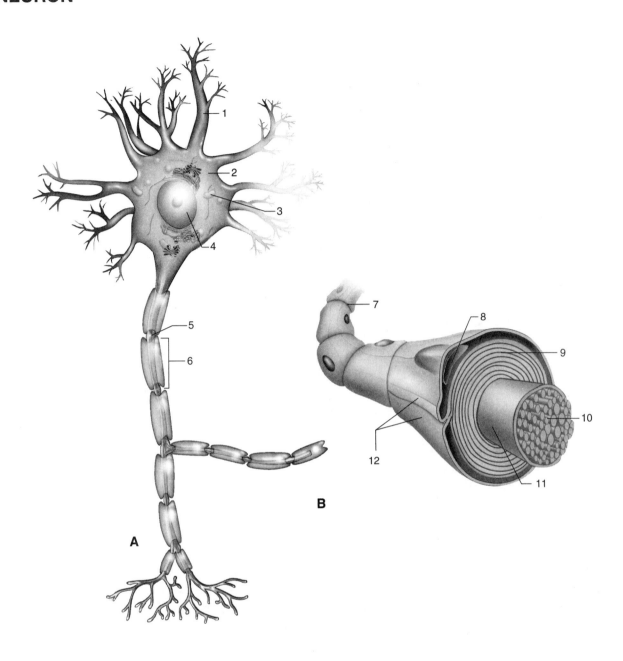

A

B

1. _____   7. _____

2. _____   8. _____

3. _____   9. _____

4. _____   10. _____

5. _____   11. _____

6. _____   12. _____

CRANIAL NERVES

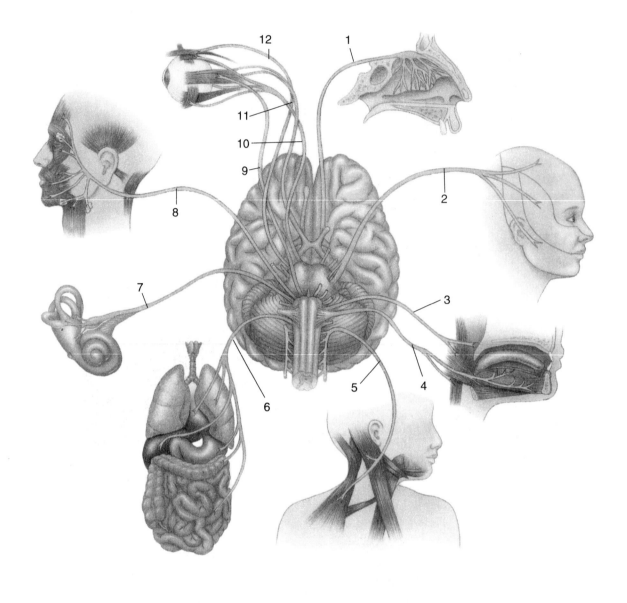

1. _____   7. _____

2. _____   8. _____

3. _____   9. _____

4. _____   10. _____

5. _____   11. _____

6. _____   12. _____

SAGITTAL SECTION OF THE CENTRAL NERVOUS SYSTEM

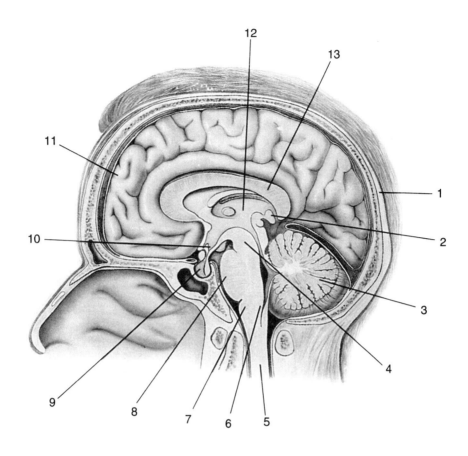

1. _____   8. _____

2. _____   9. _____

3. _____   10. _____

4. _____   11. _____

5. _____   12. _____

6. _____   13. _____

7. _____

THE CEREBRUM

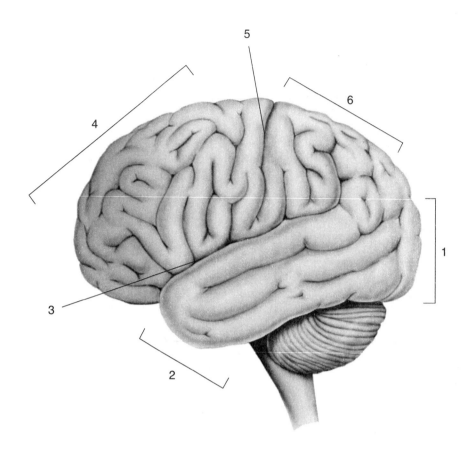

1. _____   4. _____

2. _____   5. _____

3. _____   6. _____

NEURON PATHWAYS

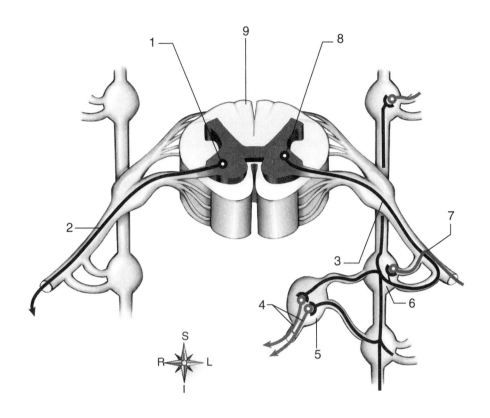

1. _____

2. _____

3. _____

4. _____

5. _____

6. _____

7. _____

8. _____

9. _____

The Senses

Consider this scene for a moment. You are walking along a beautiful beach while watching the sunset. You notice the various hues and are amazed at the multitude of shades that cover the sky. The waves are melodious as they splash along the shore, and you wiggle your feet with delight as you sense the warm, soft sand trickling between your toes. You sip on a soda and then inhale the fresh salt air as you continue your stroll along the shore. It is a memorable scene, but one that would not be possible without the assistance of your sense organs. The sense organs pick up messages that are sent over nerve pathways to specialized areas in the brain for interpretation. They make communication with and enjoyment of the environment possible. The visual, auditory, tactile, olfactory, and gustatory sense organs not only protect us from danger but also add an important dimension to our daily pleasures of life.

Your study of this chapter will give you an understanding of another one of the systems necessary for homeostasis and survival.

TOPICS FOR REVIEW

Before progressing to Chapter 11, you should review the classification of sense organs and the process for converting a stimulus into a sensation. Your study should also include an understanding of the special sense organs and the general sense organs.

CLASSIFICATION OF SENSE ORGANS
CONVERTING A STIMULUS INTO A SENSATION
GENERAL SENSE ORGANS

Match each term on the left with the corresponding description on the right.

_____ 1. Special sense organ   A. Olfactory cells

_____ 2. General sense organ   B. Detects stimuli such as pain or touch

_____ 3. Nose   C. Gustatory cells

_____ 4. Bulboid (Krause) corpuscle   D. Eye

_____ 5. Taste   E. Touch and possibly cold

▶ *If you had difficulty with this section, review pages 281-283 and Tables 10-1 and 10-2.*

SPECIAL SENSE ORGANS

Eye

Circle the correct answer.

6. The "white" of the eye is more commonly called the:
   A. Choroid
   B. Cornea
   C. Sclera
   D. Retina
   E. None of the above is correct.

7. The "colored" part of the eye is known as the:
   A. Retina
   B. Cornea
   C. Pupil
   D. Sclera
   E. Iris

8. The transparent portion of the sclera, referred to as the "window" of the eye, is the:
   A. Retina
   B. Cornea
   C. Pupil
   D. Iris

9. The mucous membrane that covers the front of the eye is called the:
   A. Cornea
   B. Choroid
   C. Conjunctiva
   D. Ciliary body
   E. None of the above is correct.

10. The structure that can contract or dilate to allow more or less light to enter the eye is the:
    A. Lens
    B. Choroid
    C. Retina
    D. Cornea
    E. Iris

11. When the eye is looking at objects far in the distance, the lens is _____ and the ciliary muscle is _____.
    A. Rounded, contracted
    B. Rounded, relaxed
    C. Slightly rounded, contracted
    D. Slightly curved, relaxed
    E. None of the above is correct

12. The lens of the eye is held in place by the:
    A. Ciliary muscle
    B. Aqueous humor
    C. Vitreous humor
    D. Cornea

13. When the lens loses its elasticity and can no longer bring near objects into focus, the condition is known as:
    A. Glaucoma
    B. Presbyopia
    C. Astigmatism
    D. Strabismus

14. The fluid in front of the lens that is constantly being formed, drained, and replaced in the anterior cavity is the:
    A. Vitreous humor
    B. Protoplasm
    C. Aqueous humor
    D. Conjunctiva

15. If drainage of the aqueous humor is blocked, the internal pressure within the eye will increase and a condition known as _____ could occur.
    A. Presbyopia
    B. Glaucoma
    C. Color blindness
    D. Cataracts

16. The rods and cones are the visual receptors and are located on the:
    A. Sclera
    B. Cornea
    C. Choroid
    D. Retina

17. Photoreception is the sense of:
    A. Vision
    B. Smell
    C. Taste
    D. Balance

18. The "blind spot" may also be referred to as the:
    A. Fovea centralis
    B. Macula lutea
    C. Retinal artery
    D. Optic disc

▶ *If you had difficulty with this section, review pages 284-288.*

Visual Disorders

Match the following terms with the numbered descriptions and write the corresponding letter in the answer blank.

A. Strabismus
B. Retinopathy
C. Myopia
D. Glaucoma
E. Astigmatism

F. Conjunctivitis
G. Nyctalopia
H. Hyperopia
I. Scotoma
J. Cataracts

_____ 19.   Nearsightedness

_____ 20.   An irregularity in the cornea

_____ 21.   "Pink-eye"

_____ 22.   "Cross-eye"

_____ 23.   Cloudy spots in the eye's lens

_____ 24.   Often caused by diabetes mellitus

_____ 25.   Farsightedness

_____ 26.   "Night blindness"

_____ 27.   Loss of only the center of the visual field

_____ 28.   Excessive intraocular pressure caused by abnormal accumulation of aqueous humor

▶ *If you had difficulty with this section, review pages 288-294.*

Ear

Match the divisions of the ear with the numbered terms and write the corresponding letter in the answer blank.

A. External ear   B. Middle ear   C. Inner ear

_____ 29.   Malleus

_____ 30.   Perilymph

_____ 31.   Incus

_____ 32.   Ceruminous glands

_____ 33.   Cochlea

_____ 34.   Acoustic canal

_____ 35.   Semicircular canals

_____ 36.   Stapes

_____ 37.   Tympanic membrane

_____ 38.   Organ of Corti

Fill in the blanks.

39. The external ear has two parts: the _____ and the

_____ _____

_____.

40. Another name for the tympanic membrane is the _____.

41. The bones of the middle ear are collectively referred to as _____.

42. The stapes presses against a membrane that covers a small opening called the

_____ _____.

43. A middle ear infection is called _____

_____.

44. The _____ is located adjacent to the oval window between the semicircular canals and the cochlea.

45. Located within the semicircular canals and the vestibule are _____ for
balance and equilibrium.

46. The sensory cells in the _____ _____
are stimulated when movement of the head causes the endolymph to move.

▶ *If you had difficulty with this section, review pages 294-298.*

Hearing Disorders

Match the terms with the numbered descriptions and write the corresponding letter in the answer blank.

A. Tinnitus   D. Otitis media
B. Presbycusis   E. Mastoiditis
C. Otosclerosis   F. Ménière disease

_____ 47.   Inherited bone disorder that impairs conduction by causing structural irregularities in the stapes

_____ 48.   "Ringing in the ear"

_____ 49.   Middle ear infection

_____ 50.   Untreated otitis media can lead to this condition

_____ 51.   Progressive hearing loss associated with aging

_____ 52.   Chronic inner ear disease characterized by progressive nerve deafness and vertigo

▶ *If you had difficulty with this section, review pages 298-299.*

TASTE RECEPTORS
SMELL RECEPTORS
GENERAL SENSE ORGANS

Circle the correct answer.

53. Structures known as (*papillae* or *olfactory cells*) are found on the tongue.

54. Nerve impulses generated by stimulation of taste buds travel primarily through two (*cranial* or *spinal*) nerves.

55. To be detected by olfactory receptors, chemicals must be dissolved in the watery (*mucus* or *plasma*) that lines the nasal cavity.

56. The pathways taken by olfactory nerve impulses and the areas where these impulses are interpreted are closely associated with areas of the brain important in (*hearing* or *memory*).

57. Receptors responsible for the sense of smell are known as (*chemoreceptors* or *mechanoreceptors*).

▶ *If you had difficulty with this section, review pages 299-302.*

UNSCRAMBLE THE WORDS

58. **C A L R I E U**

59. **R A E C L S**

60. **L A P I L A E P**

61. **C T V N U C N O I A J**

Take the circled letters, unscramble them, and fill in the solution.

What Mr. Tuttle liked best about his classroom.

62.

APPLYING WHAT YOU KNOW

63. Mr. Nay was an avid swimmer and competed regularly in his age group. He had to withdraw from the last competition due to an infection of his ear. Antibiotics and analgesics were prescribed by the doctor. What is the medical term for his condition?

64. Mrs. Metheny loved the out-of-doors and spent a great deal of her spare time basking in the sun on the beach. Her physician suggested that she begin wearing sunglasses regularly when he noticed milky spots beginning to appear on Mrs. Metheny's lenses. What condition was Mrs. Metheny's physician trying to prevent from occurring?

65. Amanda repeatedly became ill with throat infections during her first few years of school. Lately, however, she has noticed that whenever she has a throat infection, her ears become very sore also. What might be the cause of this additional problem?

66. Richard was hit in the nose with a baseball during practice. His sense of smell was temporarily gone. What nerve receptors were damaged during the injury?

67. Word Find

Find and circle 19 terms presented in this chapter. Words may be spelled top to bottom, bottom to top, right to left, left to right, or diagonally.

```
M E C H A N O R E C E P T O R
H R A T B Q I R T B N H M A E
P F T Y R O T C A F L O X R C
G U A Y I N A I H C A T S U E
G P R A C E R U M E N O P X P
I E A I P O Y B S E R P K D T
W L C P L Y N E Y K E I T O O
C Q T O I B R J B S F G L M R
Z U S R C L E O U J R M N N S
F D M E O H L Q T N A E Y I S
H I D P N D L A M A C N X S Z
A M L Y E S S E E D T T M Z H
D D M H S F E X A Y I S I I A
J C G N J T I S L P O G U V J
P H G Y A K H S U C N I S G A
```

Cataracts	Gustatory	Presbyopia
Cerumen	Hyperopia	Receptors
Cochlea	Incus	Refraction
Cones	Mechanoreceptor	Rods
Conjunctiva	Olfactory	Senses
Eustachian	Papillae	
Eye	Photopigment	

DID YOU KNOW?

Glaucoma is the leading cause of blindness among African Americans.

THE SENSES

Fill in the crossword puzzle.

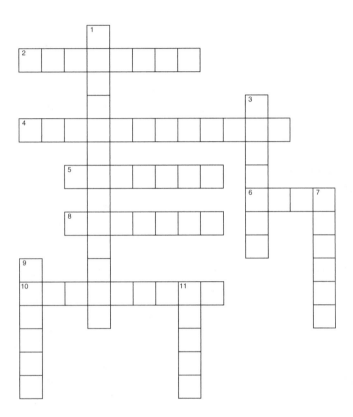

ACROSS

2. Bones of the middle ear
4. Located in anterior cavity in front of lens (two words)
5. External ear
6. Transparent body behind pupil
8. Front part of this coat is the ciliary muscle and iris
10. Membranous labyrinth filled with this fluid

DOWN

1. Located in posterior cavity (two words)
3. Organ of Corti located here
7. White of the eye
9. Innermost layer of the eye
11. Hole in center of the iris

CHECK YOUR KNOWLEDGE

Multiple Choice

Circle the correct answer.

1. Where are the specialized mechanoreceptors of hearing and balance located?
   A. Inner ear
   B. Malleus
   C. Helix
   D. All of the above

2. The organ of Corti is the organ of what sense?
   A. Sight
   B. Hearing
   C. Pressure
   D. Taste

3. Where are taste sensations interpreted?
   A. Cerebral cortex
   B. Area of stimulation
   C. Nasal cavity
   D. None of the above

4. A surgical technique to treat myopia without the use of glasses or contacts is called:
   A. Presbyopia
   B. Removal of cataracts
   C. Radial keratotomy
   D. None of the above

5. Which of the following statements about the cornea is true?
   A. It is a mucous membrane.
   B. It is called the "window of the eye."
   C. It lies behind the iris.
   D. All of the above are true.

6. Which of the following are general sense organs?
   A. Gustatory receptors
   B. Pacini corpuscles
   C. Olfactory receptors
   D. All of the above

7. The retina contains microscopic receptor cells called:
   A. Mechanoreceptors
   B. Chemoreceptors
   C. Olfactory receptors
   D. Rods and cones

8. Which two involuntary muscles make up the front part of the eye?
   A. Malleus and incus
   B. Iris and ciliary muscle
   C. Retina and pacinian muscle
   D. Sclera and iris

9. Which of the following statements about gustatory sense organs is true?
   A. They are called *taste buds*.
   B. They are innervated by cranial nerves VII and IX.
   C. They work together with the olfactory senses.
   D. All of the above are true.

10. The external ear consists of the:
    A. Auricle and acoustic canal
    B. Labyrinth
    C. Corti and cochlea
    D. None of the above

True/False

If the statement is true, write "T" in the answer blank. If the statement is false, correct the statement by circling the incorrect term and writing the correct term in the answer blank.

_____ 11. The tympanic membrane separates the middle ear from the external ear.

_____ 12. Glaucoma may result from a blockage of flow of vitreous humor.

_____ 13. With the condition of presbyopia, the eye lens loses its elasticity.

_____ 14. The bones of the middle ear are the malleus, incus, and ossicles.

_____ 15. Myopia occurs when images are focused in front of the retina rather than on it.

_____ 16. Light enters through the pupil, and the size of the pupil is regulated by the iris.

_____ 17. The retina is the innermost layer of the eye. It contains the structures called *rods*.

_____ 18. A commonly used name for the "white of the eye" is the sclera.

_____ 19. The olfactory receptors are chemical receptors.

_____ 20. The organ of Corti contains mechanoreceptors.

EYE

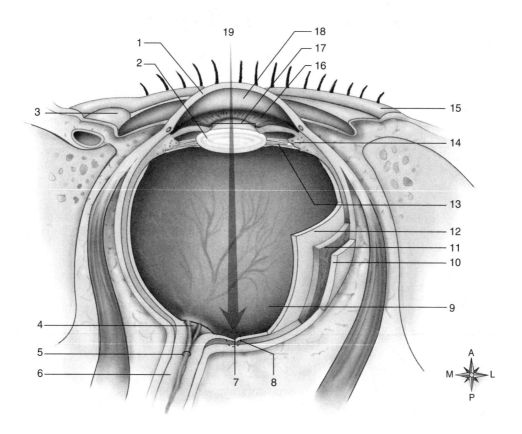

1. _____

2. _____

3. _____

4. _____

5. _____

6. _____

7. _____

8. _____

9. _____

10. _____

11. _____

12. _____

13. _____

14. _____

15. _____

16. _____

17. _____

18. _____

19. _____

EAR

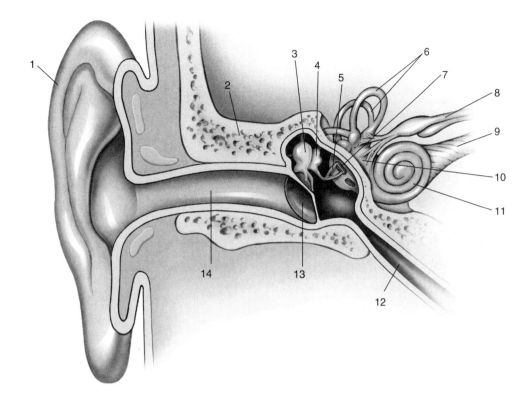

1. _____

2. _____

3. _____

4. _____

5. _____

6. _____

7. _____

8. _____

9. _____

10. _____

11. _____

12. _____

13. _____

14. _____

The Endocrine System

T he endocrine system is often compared to a fine concert symphony. When all instruments are playing properly, the sound is melodious. If one instrument plays too loud or too soft, however, it affects the overall quality of the entire performance.

The endocrine system is a ductless system that releases hormones into the bloodstream to help regulate body functions. The pituitary gland may be considered the conductor of the orchestra, because it stimulates many of the endocrine glands to secrete their powerful hormones. All hormones, whether stimulated in this manner or by other control mechanisms, are interdependent. A change in the level of one hormone may affect the level of many other hormones.

In addition to the endocrine glands, prostaglandins, or "tissue hormones," are powerful substances similar to hormones that have been found in a variety of body tissues. These hormones are often produced in a tissue and diffuse only a short distance to act on cells within that area. Prostaglandins influence respiration, blood pressure, gastrointestinal secretions, and the reproductive system and may some day play an important role in the treatment of diseases such as hypertension, asthma, and ulcers.

The endocrine system is a system of communication and control. It differs from the nervous system in that hormones provide a slower, longer-lasting effect than do nerve stimuli and responses. Your understanding of the "system of hormones" will give you a new awareness of the mechanism of our emotions, response to stress, growth, chemical balances, and many other body functions.

TOPICS FOR REVIEW

Before progressing to Chapter 12, you should be able to identify and locate the primary endocrine glands of the body. Your understanding should include the hormones that are produced by these glands and the method by which these secretions are regulated. Your study will conclude with the pathological conditions that result from the malfunction of this system.

MECHANISMS OF HORMONE ACTION
REGULATION OF HORMONE SECRETION
MECHANISMS OF ENDOCRINE DISEASE
PROSTAGLANDINS

Match each term on the left with the corresponding word or phrase on the right.

Group A

_____ 1. Pituitary
_____ 2. Parathyroids
_____ 3. Adrenals
_____ 4. Ovaries
_____ 5. Thymus

A. Pelvic cavity
B. Mediastinum
C. Neck
D. Cranial cavity
E. Abdominal cavity

Group B

_____ 6. Negative feedback

_____ 7. Tissue hormones
_____ 8. Polyendocrine disorders
_____ 9. Exocrine glands
_____ 10. Target organ cells

A. Result from hyposecretion or hypersecretion of several hormones
B. Respond to a particular hormone
C. Prostaglandins
D. Discharge secretions into ducts
E. Specialized homeostatic mechanism that regulates release of hormones

Fill in the blanks.

Nonsteroid hormones work according to the (11) _____

_____ mechanism. According to this concept, a

(12) _____ hormone acts as a (13) _____

_____, providing communication between endocrine glands and

(14) _____ _____. A second messenger,

such as (15) _____ _____, provides com-

munication within a hormone's (16) _____

_____. (17) _____

_____ disrupts the normal negative feedback control of hormones through-

out the body and may result in tissue damage, sterility, mental imbalance, and a host of life-threatening meta-

bolic problems.

▶ *If you had difficulty with this section, review pages 309-317.*

PITUITARY GLAND
HYPOTHALAMUS

Circle the correct answer.

18. The pituitary gland lies in the _____ bone.
    A. Ethmoid
    B. Sphenoid
    C. Temporal
    D. Frontal
    E. Occipital

19. Which one of the following structures would *not* be stimulated by a tropic hormone from the anterior pituitary?
    A. Ovaries
    B. Testes
    C. Thyroid
    D. Adrenals
    E. Uterus

20. Which one of the following is *not* a function of FSH?
    A. Stimulates the growth of follicles
    B. Stimulates the production of estrogens
    C. Stimulates the growth of seminiferous tubules
    D. Stimulates the interstitial cells of the testes

21. Which one of the following is *not* a function of LH?
    A. Stimulates maturation of a developing follicle
    B. Stimulates the production of estrogens
    C. Stimulates the formation of a corpus luteum
    D. Stimulates sperm cells to mature in the male
    E. Causes ovulation to occur

22. Which one of the following is *not* a function of GH?
    A. Increases glucose catabolism
    B. Increases fat catabolism
    C. Speeds up the movement of amino acids into cells from the bloodstream
    D. All of the above are functions of GH

23. Which one of the following hormones is *not* released by the anterior pituitary gland?
    A. ACTH
    B. TSH
    C. ADH
    D. FSH
    E. LH

24. Which one of the following is *not* a function of prolactin?
    A. Stimulates breast development during pregnancy
    B. Stimulates milk secretion after delivery
    C. Causes the release of milk from glandular cells of the breast
    D. All of the above are functions of prolactin

25. The anterior pituitary gland secretes:
    A. Eight major hormones
    B. Tropic hormones that stimulate other endocrine glands to grow and secrete
    C. ADH
    D. Oxytocin

26. TSH acts on the:
    A. Thyroid
    B. Thymus
    C. Pineal gland
    D. Testes

27. ACTH stimulates the:
    A. Adrenal cortex
    B. Adrenal medulla
    C. Hypothalamus
    D. Ovaries

28. Which hormone is secreted by the posterior pituitary gland?
    A. MSH
    B. LH
    C. GH
    D. ADH

29. ADH serves the body by:
    A. Initiating labor
    B. Accelerating water reabsorption from urine into the blood
    C. Stimulating the pineal gland
    D. Regulating the calcium/phosphorus levels in the blood

30. The disease caused by hyposecretion of ADH is:
    A. Diabetes insipidus
    B. Diabetes mellitus
    C. Acromegaly
    D. Myxedema

31. The actual production of ADH and oxytocin takes place in which area?
    A. Anterior pituitary
    B. Posterior pituitary
    C. Hypothalamus
    D. Pineal gland

32. Inhibiting hormones are produced by the:
    A. Anterior pituitary
    B. Posterior pituitary
    C. Hypothalamus
    D. Pineal gland

Match one of the glands listed with each numbered term and write the corresponding letter in the answer blank.

A. Anterior pituitary   B. Posterior pituitary   C. Hypothalamus

_____ 33.   Adenohypophysis

_____ 34.   Neurohypophysis

_____ 35.   Induced labor

_____ 36.   Appetite

_____ 37.   Acromegaly

_____ 38.   Body temperature

_____ 39.   Sex hormones

_____ 40.   Tropic hormones

_____ 41.   Gigantism

_____ 42.   Releasing hormones

▶ *If you had difficulty with this section, review pages 317-320 and Table 11-1.*

THYROID GLAND

PARATHYROID GLANDS

Circle the correct answer.

43. The thyroid gland lies (*above* or *below*) the larynx.

44. The thyroid gland secretes (*calcitonin* or *glucagon*).

45. For thyroxine to be produced in adequate amounts, the diet must contain sufficient (*calcium* or *iodine*).

46. Most endocrine glands (*do* or *do not*) store their hormones.

47. Colloid is a storage medium for the (*thyroid* or *parathyroid*) hormone.

48. Calcitonin (*increases* or *decreases*) the concentration of calcium in the blood.

49. A goiter results from (*hyperthyroidism* or *hypothyroidism*).

50. Hyposecretion of thyroid hormones during the formative years leads to (*cretinism* or *myxedema*).

51. The parathyroid glands secrete the hormone (*PTH* or *PTA*).

52. Parathyroid hormone tends to (*increase* or *decrease*) the concentration of calcium in the blood.

▶ *If you had difficulty with this section, review pages 320-323.*

ADRENAL GLANDS

Fill in the blanks.

53. The adrenal gland is actually two separate endocrine glands, the _____
    _____ and the _____
    _____.

54. Hormones secreted by the adrenal cortex are known as _____.

55. The outer zone of the adrenal cortex, the zona glomerulosa, secretes _____.

56. The middle zone, the zona fasciculata, secretes _____.

57. The innermost zone, the zona reticularis, secretes _____
    _____.

58. Glucocorticoids act in several ways to increase _____.

59. Glucocorticoids also play an essential part in maintaining _____
    _____.

60. The adrenal medulla secretes the hormones _____ and
    _____.

61. The adrenal glands may help the body resist _____.

62. A _____ tumor of the adrenal cortex causes masculinizing symptoms
    to appear in a woman.

Match each of numbered terms with the related adrenal structure and write the corresponding letter in the answer blank.

A. Adrenal cortex   B. Adrenal medulla

_____ 63.   Addison disease

_____ 64.   Anti-immunity

_____ 65.   Adrenaline

_____ 66.   Cushing syndrome

_____ 67.   Fight-or-flight syndrome

_____ 68.   Aldosterone

_____ 69.   Androgens

▶ *If you had difficulty with this section, review pages 323-328.*

PANCREATIC ISLETS
SEX GLANDS
THYMUS
PLACENTA
PINEAL GLAND

Circle the word in each word group that does not belong.

70. Alpha cells   Glucagon   Beta cells   Glycogenolysis

71. Insulin   Glucagon   Beta cells   Diabetes mellitus

72. Estrogens   Progesterone   Corpus luteum   Thymosin

73. Chorion   Interstitial cells   Testosterone   Semen

74. Immune system   Mediastinum   Aldosterone   Thymosin

75. Pregnancy   ACTH   Estrogen   Chorion

76. Melatonin   Sleep cycle   "Third eye"   Semen

Match each term on the left with the corresponding hormone on the right.

Group A

_____ 77. Alpha cells   A. Estrogen

_____ 78. Beta cells   B. Progesterone

_____ 79. Corpus luteum   C. Insulin

_____ 80. Interstitial cells   D. Testosterone

_____ 81. Ovarian follicles   E. Glucagon

Group B

_____ 82. Placenta   A. Melatonin

_____ 83. Pineal gland   B. ANH

_____ 84. Heart atria   C. Testosterone

_____ 85. Testes   D. Thymosin

_____ 86. Thymus   E. Chorionic gonadotropin

▶ *If you had difficulty with this section, review pages 328-332.*

UNSCRAMBLE THE WORDS

87. **R O O D I I T S C C**

□□□□□□□□□◯□

88. **S I U I S E R D**

□□□□◯◯□□

89. **U O O O T D C S I I L R C C G**

□□□□□□◯□□□□□□□

90. **R I O D S T E S**

◯□□◯□□□□

Take the circled letters, unscramble them, and fill in the solution.

Why Billy didn't like to take exams.

91. □□□□□□□

APPLYING WHAT YOU KNOW

92. Mrs. Tips made a routine visit to her physician last week. When the laboratory results came back, the report indicated a high level of chorionic gonadotropin in her urine. What did this mean to Mrs. Tips?

93. Mrs. Wilcox noticed that her daughter was beginning to take on the secondary sex characteristics of a male. The pediatrician diagnosed the condition as a tumor of an endocrine gland. Where specifically was the tumor located?

94. Mrs. Liddy was pregnant and was 2 weeks past her due date. Her doctor suggested that she enter the hospital and he would induce labor. What hormone will he give Mrs. Liddy?

95. Word Find

Find and circle 16 terms presented in this chapter. Words may be spelled top to bottom, bottom to top, right to left, left to right, or diagonally.

```
S  S  I  S  E  R  U  I  D  M  E  S  I  T  W
N  D  N  X  E  B  A  M  E  D  E  X  Y  M  I
I  I  G  O  N  R  S  G  X  T  I  I  Y  V  B
D  O  M  S  I  N  I  T  E  R  C  C  U  Q  D
N  C  X  S  R  T  N  B  O  T  V  M  Y  O  M
A  I  M  E  C  L  A  C  R  E  P  Y  H  I  X
L  T  Y  R  O  I  E  Z  Q  R  T  J  V  K  F
G  R  E  T  D  P  S  N  I  L  D  J  M  X  N
A  O  O  S  N  I  D  K  I  N  K  S  P  P  O
T  C  P  R  E  T  I  O  G  R  I  F  M  X  G
S  L  M  H  Y  P  O  G  L  Y  C  E  M  I  A
O  A  J  L  H  O  R  M  O  N  E  O  T  G  C
R  C  E  L  T  S  E  L  C  N  P  N  X  U  U
P  I  O  S  W  R  T  X  C  G  U  L  O  E  L
G  G  V  Y  H  M  S  H  Y  K  A  K  N  Q  G
```

Corticoids	Glucagon	Myxedema
Cretinism	Goiter	Prostaglandins
Diabetes	Hormone	Steroids
Diuresis	Hypercalcemia	Stress
Endocrine	Hypoglycemia	
Exocrine	Luteinization	

DID YOU KNOW?

The total daily output of the pituitary gland is less than 1/1,000,000 of a gram, yet this small amount is responsible for stimulating the majority of all endocrine functions.

THE ENDOCRINE SYSTEM

Fill in the crossword puzzle.

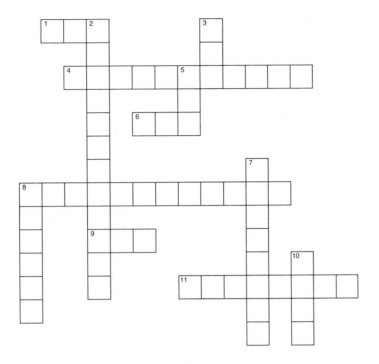

ACROSS

1. Secreted by cells in the walls of the heart's atria
4. Adrenal medulla
6. Estrogens
8. Converts amino acids to glucose
9. Melanin
11. Labor

DOWN

2. Hypersecretion of insulin
3. Antagonist to diuresis
5. Increases calcium concentration
7. Hyposecretion of islets of Langerhans (one word)
8. Hyposecretion of thyroid
10. Adrenal cortex

CHECK YOUR KNOWLEDGE

Multiple Choice

Circle the correct answer.

1. What does the outer zone of the adrenal cortex secrete?
   A. Mineralocorticoids
   B. Sex hormones
   C. Glucocorticoids
   D. Epinephrine

2. From what condition does diabetes insipidus result?
   A. Low insulin levels
   B. High glucagon levels
   C. Low antidiuretic hormone levels
   D. High steroid levels

3. Which of the following statements is true regarding a young child whose growth is stunted, metabolism is low, sexual development is delayed, and mental development is retarded?
   A. The child suffers from cretinism.
   B. The child has an underactive thyroid.
   C. The child could suffer from a pituitary disorder.
   D. All of the above are true.

4. What can result when too much growth hormone is produced by the pituitary gland?
   A. Hyperglycemia
   B. A pituitary giant
   C. Both A and B
   D. None of the above

5. Which of the following glands is *not* regulated by the pituitary?
   A. Thyroid
   B. Ovaries
   C. Adrenals
   D. Thymus

6. Which of the following statements about the antidiuretic hormone is true?
   A. It is released by the posterior lobe of the pituitary.
   B. It causes diabetes insipidus when produced in insufficient amounts.
   C. It decreases urine volume.
   D. All of the above are true.

7. What controls the development of the body's immune system?
   A. Pituitary
   B. Thymus
   C. Pineal body
   D. Thyroid

8. Administration of what would best treat a person suffering from severe allergies?
   A. Gonadocorticoids
   B. Glucagon
   C. Mineralocorticoids
   D. Glucocorticoids

9. What endocrine gland is composed of cell clusters called the *islets of Langerhans*?
   A. Adrenals
   B. Thyroid
   C. Pituitary
   D. Pancreas

10. Which of the following statements concerning prostaglandins is true?
    A. They control activities of widely separated organs.
    B. They can be called *tissue hormones*.
    C. They diffuse over long distances to act on cells.
    D. All of the above are true.

Matching

Match each term in column A with the corresponding hormone in column B. (Only one answer is correct for each.)

Column A

_____ 11. Goiter

_____ 12. Ovulation

_____ 13. Diabetes mellitus

_____ 14. Lactation

_____ 15. Diabetes insipidus

_____ 16. Chorionic gonadotropins

_____ 17. Cushing syndrome

_____ 18. Labor

_____ 19. Acromegaly

_____ 20. Hypercalcemia

Column B

A. Glucocorticoid hormones

B. Antidiuretic hormone

C. Calcitonin

D. Oxytocin

E. Growth hormone

F. Placenta

G. Luteinizing hormone

H. Insulin

I. Prolactin

J. Thyroid hormones

ENDOCRINE GLANDS

1. _____

2. _____

3. _____

4. _____

5. _____

6. _____

7. _____

8. _____

9. _____

10. _____

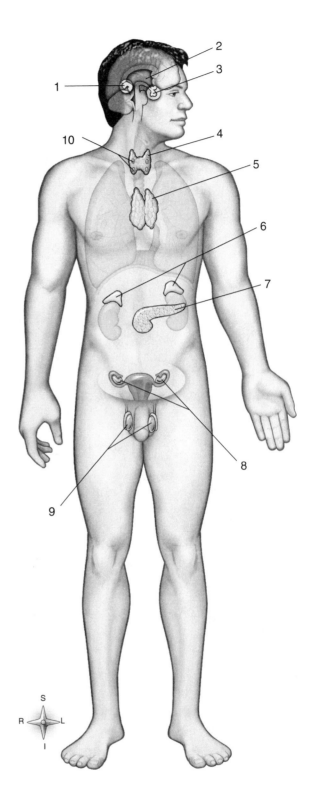

CHAPTER 12

Blood

B lood, the river of life, is the body's primary means of internal transportation. Although it is the respiratory system that provides oxygen for the body, the digestive system that provides nutrients, and the urinary system that eliminates wastes, none of these functions could be provided for the individual cells without blood. In less than 1 minute, a drop of blood will complete a trip through the entire body, distributing nutrients and collecting the wastes of metabolism.

Blood is divided into plasma (the liquid portion of blood) and the formed elements (the blood cells). There are three types of blood cells: red blood cells, white blood cells, and platelets. Together these cells and plasma provide a means of transportation that delivers the body's daily necessities.

Although all of us have red blood cells that are similar in shape, we have different blood types. Blood types are identified by the presence of certain antigens in the red blood cells. Every person's blood belongs to one of four main blood groups: Type A, B, AB, or O. Any one of the four groups or "types" may or may not have the Rh factor present in the red blood cells. If an individual has a specific antigen called the Rh factor present in his or her blood, the blood is Rh positive. If this factor is missing, the blood is Rh negative. Approximately 85% of the population has the Rh factor (Rh positive), whereas 15% do not have the Rh factor (Rh negative).

Your understanding of this chapter will be necessary to prepare a proper foundation for learning about the circulatory system.

TOPICS FOR REVIEW

Before progressing to Chapter 13, you should have an understanding of the structure and function of blood plasma and cells. Your review should also include an understanding of blood types and Rh factors.

BLOOD COMPOSITION

Circle the correct answer.

1. Which one of the following substances is *not* a part of the plasma?
   A. Water
   B. Proteins
   C. Nutrients
   D. Waste products
   E. Formed elements

2. The normal volume of blood in an adult is approximately:
   A. 2-3 pints
   B. 2-3 quarts
   C. 2-3 gallons
   D. 4-6 liters

3. Blood is normally:
   A. Very acidic
   B. Slightly acidic
   C. Neutral
   D. Slightly alkaline

4. PolyHeme is a/an:
   A. Artificial blood
   B. Antigen
   C. Antibody
   D. Plasma volume expander

5. Donated blood:
   A. Must be "typed and cross matched"
   B. Can be stored for only 6 weeks
   C. Is most valuable during the "golden hour"
   D. All of the above

   ▶ *If you had difficulty with this section, review pages 341-343.*

BLOOD TYPES

6. Fill in the blank areas.

Blood Type	Antigen Present in RBC	Antibody Present in Plasma
A	A	Anti-B
B	B	Anti A
AB	AB	None
O	None	AB

Fill in the blanks.

7. An _____ antigen _____ is a substance that can stimulate the body to make antibodies.

8. An _____ is a substance made by the body in response to stimulation by an antigen.

9. Many antibodies react with their antigens to clump or _____ coagulate _____ them.

10. If a baby is born to an Rh-negative mother and Rh-positive father, it may develop the disease _____ erythroblastosis fetalis _____.

11. The term "Rh" is used because the antigen was first discovered in the blood of a _____ monkey monkey _____.

12. The universal donor blood is _____ Type O _____.

13. The universal recipient blood is _____ Type AB _____.

▶ *If you had difficulty with this section, review pages 343-345.*

BLOOD PLASMA AND FORMED ELEMENTS

Circle the correct answer.

14. Another name for white blood cells is:
    A. Erythrocytes
    B. Leukocytes
    C. Thrombocytes
    D. Platelets

15. Another name for platelets is:
    A. Neutrophils
    B. Eosinophils
    C. Thrombocytes
    D. Erythrocytes

16. Pernicious anemia is caused by:
    A. A lack of vitamin B_{12}
    B. Hemorrhage
    C. Radiation
    D. Bleeding ulcers

17. The laboratory test called *hematocrit* tells the physician the volume of:
    A. White cells in a blood sample
    B. Red cells in a blood sample
    C. Platelets in a blood sample
    D. Plasma in a blood sample

18. An example of a nongranular leukocyte is a/an:
    A. Platelet
    B. Erythrocyte
    C. Eosinophil
    D. Monocyte

19. An excess of red blood cells is known as:
    A. Erythropenia
    B. Erythroplasia
    C. Polycythemia
    D. Anemia

20. A critical component of hemoglobin is:
    A. Potassium
    B. Calcium
    C. Vitamin K
    D. Iron

21. Sickle cell anemia is caused by:
    A. The production of an abnormal type of hemoglobin
    B. The production of excessive neutrophils
    C. The production of excessive platelets
    D. The production of abnormal leukocytes

22. The practice of using blood transfusions to increase oxygen delivery to muscles during athletic events is called:
    A. Blood antigen
    B. Blood doping
    C. Blood agglutination
    D. Blood proofing

23. One of the most useful and frequently performed clinical blood tests is called the:
    A. WBC
    B. CBC
    C. RBC
    D. Hematocrit

24. Which one of the following types of cells is not a granular leukocyte?
    A. Neutrophil
    B. Monocyte
    C. Basophil
    D. Eosinophil

25. If a blood cell has no nucleus and is shaped like a biconcave disc, then the cell most likely is a/an:
    A. Platelet
    B. Lymphocyte
    C. Basophil
    D. Eosinophil
    E. Red blood cell

26. Red bone marrow forms all kinds of blood cells except some:
    A. Platelets and basophils
    B. Lymphocytes and monocytes
    C. Red blood cells
    D. Neutrophils and eosinophils

27. Myeloid tissue is found in all but which one of the following locations?
    A. Sternum
    B. Ribs
    C. Wrist bones
    D. Hip bones
    E. Cranial bones

28. Lymphatic tissue is found in which of the following locations?
    A. Lymph nodes
    B. Thymus
    C. Spleen
    D. All of the above contain lymphatic tissue.

29. The "buffy coat" layer in a hematocrit tube contains:
    A. Red blood cells and platelets
    B. Plasma only
    C. Platelets only
    D. White blood cells and platelets
    E. None of the above is correct.

30. The hematocrit value for red blood cells is _____%.
    A. 75
    B. 60
    C. 50
    D. 45
    E. 35

31. An unusually low white blood cell count would be termed:
    A. Leukemia
    B. Leukopenia
    C. Leukocytosis
    D. Anemia
    E. None of the above is correct.

32. Most of the oxygen transported in the blood is carried by:
    A. Platelets
    B. Plasma
    C. White blood cells
    D. Red blood cells
    E. None of the above is correct.

33. The most numerous of the phagocytes are the _____.
    A. Lymphocytes
    B. Neutrophils
    C. Basophils
    D. Eosinophils
    E. Monocytes

34. Which one of the following types of cells is *not* phagocytic?
    A. Neutrophils
    B. Eosinophils
    C. Lymphocytes
    D. Monocytes
    E. All of the above are phagocytic cells.

35. Which of the following cell types functions in the immune process?
    A. Neutrophils
    B. Lymphocytes
    C. Monocytes
    D. Basophils
    E. Reticuloendothelial cells

36. Vitamin K stimulates liver cells to increase the synthesis of:
    A. Prothrombin
    B. Thrombin
    C. Platelets
    D. Heparin
    E. Calcium

37. If part of a clot dislodges and circulates through the bloodstream, the dislodged part is called a/an:
    A. Thrombus
    B. Thrombosis
    C. Anticoagulant
    D. Clotting factor
    E. Embolus

38. This disease usually occurs as a result of the destruction of bone marrow by toxic chemicals or radiation.
    A. Folate-deficiency anemia
    B. Aplastic anemia
    C. Hemolytic anemia
    D. Sickle cell anemia

39. An example of a hemolytic anemia is:
    A. Folate-deficiency anemia
    B. Aplastic anemia
    C. Sickle cell anemia
    D. Pernicious anemia

40. The disease that results from a failure to form blood clotting factor VIII is:
    A. Hemophilia
    B. Thrombocytopenia
    C. Thrombophlebitis
    D. None of the above

41. A special type of white blood cell count used as a diagnostic tool is known as a/an:
    A. Leukopenia
    B. Granulocyte count
    C. Differential WBC count
    D. CBC

▶ *If you had difficulty with this section, review pages 345-364.*

APPLYING WHAT YOU KNOW

42. Mrs. Florez's blood type is O positive. Her husband's type is O negative. Her newborn baby's blood type is O negative. Is there any need for concern with this combination?

43. After Mrs. Freund's baby was born, the doctor applied a gauze dressing for a short time on the umbilical cord. He also gave the baby a dose of vitamin K. Why did the doctor perform these two procedures?

44. Valerie was a teenager with a picky appetite. She loved junk food and seldom ate properly. She complained of being tired all the time. A visit to her doctor revealed a hemoglobin of 10 and RBCs that are classified as hypochromic. What condition does Valerie have?

45.   Word Find

Find and circle 24 terms presented in this chapter. Words may be spelled top to bottom, bottom to top, right to left, left to right, or diagonally.

```
H  S  H  K  L  S  U  L  O  B  M  E  A  E  S
K  E  E  V  M  Z  H  E  P  A  R  I  N  D  N
D  T  M  F  A  C  T  O  R  Y  E  T  I  Q  P
O  Y  A  O  H  N  B  A  T  Q  Y  A  R  A  R
N  C  T  J  G  W  E  H  N  P  N  L  B  U  D
O  O  O  S  Q  L  R  M  E  T  I  S  I  P  M
R  K  C  E  M  O  O  N  I  H  I  Q  F  W  W
H  U  R  T  C  N  I  B  P  A  S  G  Z  T  G
E  E  I  Y  O  B  O  O  I  V  E  W  E  T  X
S  L  T  C  M  D  S  E  C  N  R  T  U  N  R
U  E  Y  O  Y  A  I  M  E  K  U  E  L  Y  S
S  T  R  G  B  S  T  H  R  O  M  B  U  S  Q
E  H  Z  A  M  S  A  L  P  N  D  Z  P  O  N
T  E  N  H  F  P  D  A  P  M  E  E  I  B  W
E  W  B  P  H  K  B  O  N  C  K  W  X  V  J
```

AIDS	Factor	Phagocytes
Anemia	Fibrin	Plasma
Antibody	Hematocrit	Recipient
Antigen	Hemoglobin	Rhesus
Basophil	Heparin	Serum
Donor	Leukemia	Thrombin
Embolus	Leukocytes	Thrombus
Erythrocytes	Monocyte	Type

BLOOD

Fill in the crossword puzzle.

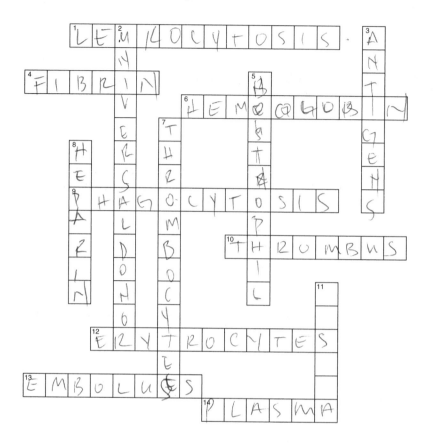

ACROSS

1. Abnormally high WBC count
4. Final stage of clotting process
6. Oxygen-carrying mechanism of blood
9. To engulf and digest microbes
10. Stationary blood clot
12. RBC
13. Circulating blood clot
14. Liquid portion of blood

DOWN

2. Type O (two words)
3. Substances that stimulate the body to make antibodies
5. Type of leukocyte
7. Platelets
8. Prevents clotting of blood
11. Inability of the blood to carry sufficient oxygen

DID YOU KNOW?

Blood products are good for approximately 3 to 6 weeks, but fresh frozen plasma is good for at least 6 months.

CHECK YOUR KNOWLEDGE

Multiple Choice

Circle the correct answer.

1. Which of the following statements is false?
   A. Sickle cell anemia is caused by a genetic defect.
   B. Leukemia is characterized by a low number of WBCs.
   C. Polycythemia is characterized by an abnormally high number of erythrocytes.
   D. Pernicious anemia is caused by a lack of vitamin B$_{12}$.

2. Deficiency in the number or function of erythrocytes is called:
   A. Leukemia
   B. Anemia
   C. Polycythemia
   D. Leukopenia

3. Which of the following statements does *not* describe a characteristic of leukocytes?
   A. They are disk-shaped cells that do not contain a nucleus.
   B. They have the ability to fight infection.
   C. They provide defense against certain parasites.
   D. They provide immune defense.

4. Which of the following substances is *not* found in serum?
   A. Clotting factors
   B. Water
   C. Hormones
   D. All of the above substances are found in serum.

5. Which of the following substances is *not* found in blood plasma?
   A. Albumins
   B. Gases
   C. Waste products
   D. All of the above substances are found in blood plasma.

6. An allergic reaction may increase the number of:
   A. Eosinophils
   B. Neutrophils
   C. Lymphocytes
   D. Monocytes

7. What is a blood clot that is moving through the body called?
   A. Embolism
   B. Fibrosis
   C. Heparin
   D. Thrombosis

8. When could difficulty with the Rh blood factor arise?
   A. When an Rh-negative man and woman produce a child.
   B. When an Rh-positive man and woman produce a child.
   C. When an Rh-positive woman and an Rh-negative man produce a child.
   D. When an Rh-negative woman and an Rh-positive man produce a child.

9. What is the primary function of hemoglobin?
   A. To fight infection
   B. To make blood clots
   C. To carry oxygen
   D. To transport hormones

10. Which of the following steps are *not* involved in blood clot formation?
    A. A blood vessel is injured and platelet factors are formed.
    B. Thrombin is converted into prothrombin.
    C. Fibrinogen is converted into fibrin.
    D. All of the above are involved in blood clot formation.

Matching

Match each term in column A with its corresponding term or description in column B. (Only one answer is correct for each.)

Column A

___D_ 11. Lymphocytes
___F_ 12. Erythrocytes
___H_ 13. Type AB
_A L_ 14. Basophils
___G_ 15. Leukemia
_C_ _A_ 16. Platelets
___B_ 17. Type O
___E_ 18. Rh factor
___I_ 19. Red bone marrow
___J_ 20. Neutrophils

Column B

A. Heparin
B. Contains anti-A and anti-B antibodies
C. Clotting
D. Immunity
E. Erythroblastosis fetalis
F. Anemia
G. Cancer
H. Contains A and B antigens
I. Myeloid tissue
J. Phagocytosis

HUMAN BLOOD CELLS

Fill in the missing areas of the table.

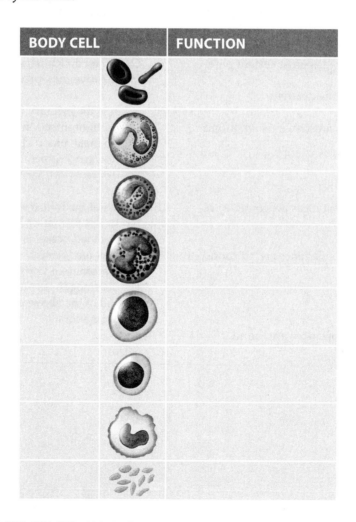

BODY CELL	FUNCTION

BLOOD TYPING

Using the key below, draw the appropriate reaction with the donor's blood in the circles.

Recipient's blood		Reactions with donor's blood			
RBC antigens	Plasma antibodies	Donor type O	Donor type A	Donor type B	Donor type AB
None (Type O)	Anti-A Anti-B	◯	◯	◯	◯
A (Type A)	Anti-B	◯	◯	◯	◯
B (Type B)	Anti-A	◯	◯	◯	◯
AB (Type AB)	(none)	◯	◯	◯	◯

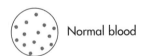 Normal blood   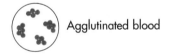 Agglutinated blood

CHAPTER 13

The Heart and Heart Disease

The heart is actually two pumps—one moves blood to the lungs, the other pushes it out into the body. These two functions seem rather elementary in comparison to the complex and numerous functions performed by most of the other body organs, and yet if this pump stops, within a few short minutes all life ceases.

The heart is divided into two upper compartments called *atria,* or receiving chambers, and two lower compartments, or discharging chambers, called *ventricles.* By age 45, approximately 300,000 tons of blood will have passed through these chambers to be circulated to the blood vessels. This closed system of circulation provides distribution of blood to the entire body (systemic circulation) and to specific regions, such as the pulmonary circulation or coronary circulation.

The beating of the heart must be coordinated in a rhythmic manner if the heart is to pump effectively. This is achieved by electrical impulses that are stimulated by specialized structures embedded in the walls of the heart. The sinoatrial node, atrioventricular node, bundle of His, and Purkinje fibers combine efforts to conduct the tiny electrical currents necessary to contract the heart. Any interruption or failure of this system may result in serious pathology or death.

A healthy heart is necessary to pump sufficient blood throughout the body to nourish and oxygenate cells continuously. Your review of this chapter will provide you with an understanding of this vital organ that is necessary for survival.

TOPICS FOR REVIEW

Before progressing to Chapter 14, you should have an understanding of the structure and function of the heart. Your review should include a study of the coronary circulation and the conduction system of the heart. Your study should conclude with an understanding of the major coronary diseases and disorders.

LOCATION, SIZE, AND POSITION OF THE HEART

ANATOMY OF THE HEART

Fill in the blanks.

1. The system that supplies our cells' transportation needs is the

   _____ _____ .

2. The _____ or blunt point at the lower edge of the heart lies on the diaphragm, pointing to the left.

3. The ___*intraventricular*___ ___*septum*___ divides the heart into right and left sides between the atria.

4. The ___*atriums*___ are the two upper chambers of the heart.

5. The ___*ventricles*___ are the two lower chambers of the heart.

6. The cardiac muscle tissue is referred to as the ___*myocardium*___.

7. Inflammation of the heart lining is ___~~pericarditis~~ *endocarditis*___.

8. The two AV valves are ___*tricuspid*___ and ___*bicuspid*___.

9. The inner layer of the pericardium is called the ___*visceral pericardium*___ or ___*epicardium*___.

10. The outer layer of pericardium is called ___*parietal pericardium*___.

11. If the pericardium becomes inflamed, a condition called ___*pericarditis*___ results.

12. The ___*semilunar*___ ___*valves*___ are located between the two ventricular chambers and the large arteries that carry blood away from the heart when contraction occurs.

13. A ___~~myocardia~~ *mitral*___ ___*valve prolapse*___ is a condition caused when the flaps of this valve extend back into the left atrium, causing the valve to leak.

14. ___~~rheumatord~~ *rheumatic* *heart disease*___ is cardiac damage resulting from a delayed inflammatory response to a streptococcal infection that occurs most often in children.

▷ *If you had difficulty with this section, review pages 373-379.*

HEART SOUNDS
BLOOD FLOW THROUGH THE HEART
CORONARY CIRCULATION AND CORONARY HEART DISEASE
HEART FAILURE

Select the term that best matches each of the numbered descriptions. Write the corresponding letter in the answer blank.

___F___ 15. Movement of blood from the left ventricle through the body

___C___ 16. Blood clot

___D___ 17. Myocardial infarction

___A___ 18. Abnormal heart sound often caused by disorders of the valves

___B___ 19. Movement of blood from the right ventricle to the lungs

___G___ 20. Hardening of the arteries

___E___ 21. Severe chest pain

___H___ 22. High blood pressure

___J___ 23. Structures through which blood returns to the left atrium

___I___ 24. Treatment for certain coronary disorders

A. ~~Heart murmur~~

B. ~~Pulmonary circulation~~

C. ~~Embolism~~

D. ~~Heart attack~~

E. ~~Angina pectoris~~

F. ~~Systemic circulation~~

G. ~~Atherosclerosis~~

H. ~~Hypertension~~

I. ~~Coronary bypass~~

J. ~~Pulmonary veins~~

CARDIAC CYCLE

CONDUCTION SYSTEM OF THE HEART

Circle the correct answer.

25. The heart beats at an average rate of _____ beats per minute.
    A. 50
    B. 72
    C. 100
    D. 120

26. Each complete beat of the heart is called:
    A. Cardiac output
    B. Stroke volume
    C. A cardiac cycle
    D. A contraction

27. The pacemaker of the heart is also known as the:
    A. SA node
    B. AV node
    C. AV bundle
    D. Purkinje fibers

28. A rapid heart rhythm, over 100 beats per minutes, is referred to as:
    A. Bradycardia
    B. Sinus arrhythmia
    C. Tachycardia
    D. Premature contractions

29. The term _____ describes the electrical activity that triggers contraction of the heart muscle.
    A. Depolarization
    B. Repolarization
    C. AV node block
    D. Cardiac arrhythmia

30. A diagnostic tool that uses ultrasound to detect valve and heart disorders is known as a/an:
    A. Electrocardiogram
    B. Pacemaker
    C. TPA
    D. Echocardiogram

31. Frequent premature contractions can lead to:
    A. Extra systoles
    B. Bradycardia
    C. Fibrillation
    D. Heart failure

32. A drug that slows and increases the strength of cardiac contractions is:
    A. Digitalis
    B. Nitroglycerin
    C. Calcium-channel blocker
    D. Anticoagulant

33. Congestive heart failure inevitably causes:
    A. Extra systole
    B. Pulmonary edema
    C. Fibrillation
    D. Bradycardia

34. Failure of the right side of the heart due to blockage of pulmonary blood flow is called:
    A. Cardiomyopathy
    B. Ventricular fibrillation
    C. Cor pulmonale
    D. TPA

35. A nonmedical rescuer can defibrillate a victim in ventricular fibrillation with the use of a/an:
    A. AED
    B. Beta-blocker
    C. Demand pacemaker
    D. ECG

36. Coumadin and dicumarol are examples of commonly used oral:
    A. Beta-blockers
    B. Nitroglycerines
    C. Calcium-channel blockers
    D. Anticoagulants

▷ *If you had difficulty with this section review pages 379-389.*

UNSCRAMBLE THE WORDS

37. **C T S S Y M E I**

S Y S T E M I C

38. **L M T R I A**

39. **T H R E A**

H E A R T

40. **S B T U M H O R**

Take the circled letters, unscramble them, and fill in the solution.

What Tom lacked on the dance floor.

41.

APPLYING WHAT YOU KNOW

42. Else was experiencing angina pectoris. Her doctor suggested a surgical procedure that would require the removal of a vein from another region of her body, which would then be used to bypass a partial blockage in her coronary arteries. What is this procedure called?

43. Phil has a heart block. His electrical impulses are being blocked and prevented from reaching the ventricles. An electrical device that causes ventricular contractions at a rate necessary to maintain circulation is being considered as possible treatment for his condition. What is this device?

44. Mrs. Haygood was diagnosed with an acute case of endocarditis. What is the real danger of this diagnosis?

45. Jeanne's homework assignment was to demonstrate knowledge of the path of blood flow through the heart. Can you help her?

Trace the blood flow through the heart by numbering the following structures in the correct sequence. Start with number 1, the vena cava, where blood enters the heart, and proceed until you have numbered all 12 structures.

2	Tricuspid valve	5	Pulmonary veins
10	Pulmonary arteries	4	Pulmonary semilunar valve
7	Bicuspid valve	7	Left ventricle
11	Vena cava	1	Right atrium
3	Right ventricle	6	Left atrium
9	Aorta	8	Aortic semilunar valve

46.   Word Find

Find and circle 12 terms presented in this chapter. Words may be spelled top to bottom, bottom to top, right to left, left to right, or diagonally.

```
P  W  S  T  L  W  G  V  F  V  W  Q  U  S  Y
U  T  X  U  L  Q  L  V  M  J  W  O  U  J  D
R  E  S  P  E  B  S  W  Z  W  K  N  X  Q  Y
K  V  Y  T  E  V  E  N  T  R  I  C  L  E  S
I  F  K  U  O  E  L  O  T  S  Y  S  X  V  R
N  G  Z  O  A  R  G  A  Y  C  M  X  F  K  H
J  B  B  C  U  J  T  R  V  K  P  Y  P  W  Y
E  V  L  A  V  R  A  N  U  L  I  M  E  S  T
F  D  T  I  Z  N  H  I  Y  A  A  D  U  T  H
I  T  B  D  O  D  S  H  Y  P  U  R  W  I  M
B  P  E  R  I  C  A  R  D  I  U  M  T  D  I
E  M  O  A  B  R  A  D  Y  C  A  R  D  I  A
R  C  U  C  E  N  D  O  C  A  R  D  I  U  M
S  A  I  D  R  A  C  Y  H  C  A  T  B  Y  P
```

Bradycardia   Endocardium   Semilunar valve
Cardiac output   Mitral valve   Systole
Coronary sinus   Pericardium   Tachycardia
Dysrhythmia   Purkinje fibers   Ventricle

DID YOU KNOW?

Your heart pumps more than 5 quarts of blood every minute—that's 2,000 gallons a day!

HEART AND HEART DISEASE

Fill in the crossword puzzle.

ACROSS

1. Inflammation of the pericardium
3. A condition in which muscle fibers contract out of step with each other
6. Disease of the myocardial tissue
8. Also known as the *visceral pericardium*
9. Relaxation of the heart
10. Upper chambers of the heart

DOWN

2. Heart specialist
4. Also known as the *sinoatrial node*
5. Complex that occurs as a result of depolarization of the ventricles
7. Also known as the *mitral valve*
8. Graphic record of the heart's electrical activity

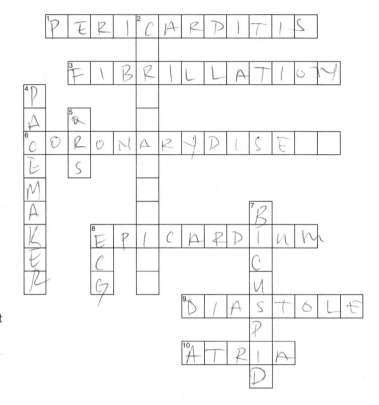

CHECK YOUR KNOWLEDGE

Multiple Choice

Circle the correct answer.

1. The superior vena cava carries blood to the:
   A. Left ventricle
   B. Coronary arteries
   C. Right atrium
   D. Pulmonary veins

2. Which of the following events, if any, does *not* precede ventricular contraction?
   A. P wave
   B. Atrial depolarization
   C. Ventricular depolarization
   D. All of these events precede contraction.

3. Which of the following pairs is mismatched?
   A. Angina pectoris—chest pain
   B. Congestive heart failure—left-sided heart failure
   C. Tachycardia—slow heart rhythm
   D. Dysrhythmia—heart block

4. Which of the following statements is *not* true regarding pericarditis?
   A. It may be caused by infection or trauma.
   B. It often causes severe chest pain.
   C. It may result in impairment of the pumping action of the heart.
   D. All of the above statements are true.

5. The outside covering that surrounds and protects the heart is called the:
   - A. Endocardium
   - B. Myocardium
   - C. Pericardium
   - D. Ectocardium

6. Thin-walled upper heart cavities that receive blood from veins are called:
   - A. Chordae tendineae
   - B. Atria
   - C. Pericardia
   - D. Ventricles

7. A valve that permits blood to flow from the right ventricle into the pulmonary artery is called:
   - A. Tricuspid
   - B. Mitral
   - C. Aortic semilunar
   - D. Pulmonary semilunar

8. Ventricular contraction of the heart occurs *immediately after* depolarization of the:
   - A. Purkinje fibers
   - B. Atrioventricular node
   - C. Sinoatrial node
   - D. Bundle of His

9. A variation in heart rate during the breathing cycle is called:
   - A. Mitral valve prolapse
   - B. Fibrillation
   - C. Sinus dysrhythmia
   - D. None of the above

10. Heart implants:
    - A. Allow patients to move around freely without external pumps.
    - B. Are artificial hearts that are made of biologically inert synthetic materials.
    - C. Weigh approximately 2 pounds.
    - D. All of the above are true.

Matching

Match each term in column A with its corresponding term in column B. (Only one answer is correct for each.)

Column A

- F 11. Heart attack
- D 12. QRS complex
- H 13. Systole
- I 14. Pulmonary circulation
- J 15. Bicuspid
- B 16. Heart compression
- C 17. Heart muscle
- A 18. Pacemaker
- G 19. T wave
- E 20. Chest pain

Column B

- A. Sinoatrial node
- B. Cardiac tamponade
- C. Myocardium
- D. Ventricular repolarization
- E. Angina pectoris
- F. Myocardial infarction
- G. Ventricular depolarization
- H. Ventricular contraction
- I. Lungs
- J. Mitral

THE HEART

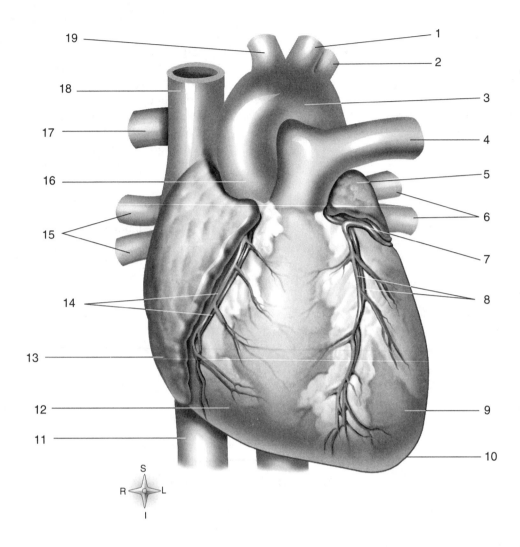

1. _____

2. _____

3. _____

4. _____

5. _____

6. _____

7. _____

8. _____

9. _____

10. _____

11. _____

12. _____

13. _____

14. _____

15. _____

16. _____

17. _____

18. _____

19. _____

CONDUCTION SYSTEM OF THE HEART

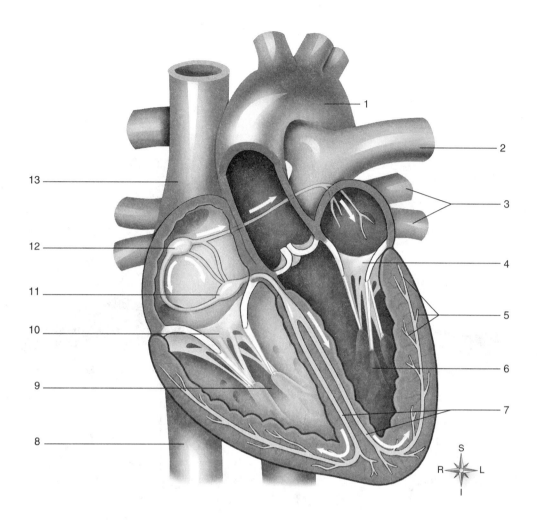

1. _aorta_
2. _pulmonary artery_
3. _pulmonary artery veins_
4. _bicuspid valve_
5. _purkinje fibers_
6. _left ventricle_
7. _AV bundles_
8. _inferior vena cava_
9. _tricuspid right ventricle_
10. _tricuspid_
11. _AV node_
12. _SA node_
13. _superior vena cava_

NORMAL ECG DEFLECTIONS

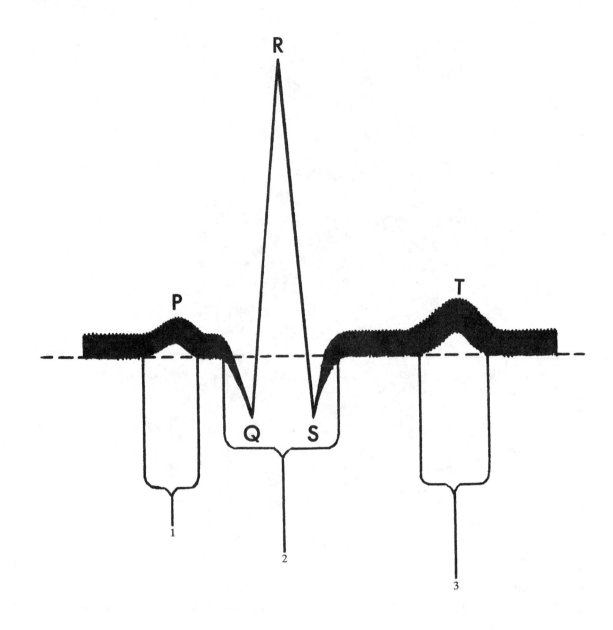

1. _____   3. _____

2. _____

CHAPTER 14

The Circulation of the Blood

O ne hundred thousand miles of blood vessels make up the elaborate transportation system that circulates materials needed for energy, growth and repair, and also eliminates wastes from your body. These vessels, called *arteries, veins,* and *capillaries,* serve different functions. Arteries carry blood from the heart, veins carry blood to the heart, and capillaries are exchange vessels, or connecting links, between the arteries and veins. The pumping action of the heart keeps blood moving, or circulating, through this closed system of vessels. This system provides distribution of blood to the entire body (systemic circulation) and to specific regions such as the pulmonary circulation or hepatic portal circulation.

Blood pressure is the force of blood in the vessels. This force is highest in the arteries and lowest in the veins. Normal blood pressure varies among individuals and depends on the volume of blood in the arteries. The larger the volume of blood in the arteries, the more pressure is exerted on the walls of the arteries, and the higher the arterial pressure. Conversely, the less blood in the arteries, the lower the blood pressure.

A functional cardiovascular system is vital for survival because without circulation, tissues would lack a supply of oxygen and nutrients. Waste products would begin to accumulate and could become toxic. Your review of this system will provide you with an understanding of the complex transportation mechanism of the body necessary for survival.

TOPICS FOR REVIEW

Before progressing to Chapter 15, you should have an understanding of the structure and function of the blood vessels. Your review should include a study of systemic, pulmonary, hepatic portal, and fetal circulation and should conclude with a thorough understanding of blood pressure, pulse, and circulatory shock.

BLOOD VESSELS

Match each term on the left with its corresponding description on the right.

_____ 1.	Arteries	A.	Smooth muscle cells that guard the entrance to capillaries
_____ 2.	Veins	B.	Carry blood to the heart
_____ 3.	Capillaries	C.	Carry blood into the venules
_____ 4.	Tunica externa	D.	Carry blood away from the heart
_____ 5.	Precapillary sphincters	E.	Largest vein
_____ 6.	Superior vena cava	F.	Largest artery
_____ 7.	Aorta	G.	Outermost layer of arteries and veins

▶ *If you had difficulty with this section, review pages 395-400.*

DISORDERS OF BLOOD VESSELS

Match each definition on the left with its corresponding term on the right.

_____ 8.	Hardening of the arteries	A.	Atherosclerosis
_____ 9.	Decreased blood supply to a tissue	B.	Ischemia
_____ 10.	Tissue death	C.	Aneurysm
_____ 11.	Necrosis that has progressed to decay	D.	Necrosis
_____ 12.	A type of arteriosclerosis caused by lipids	E.	Gangrene
_____ 13.	A section of an artery that has become abnormally widened	F.	Hemorrhoids
_____ 14.	Varicose veins in the rectum	G.	Phlebitis
_____ 15.	Vein inflammation	H.	Stroke
_____ 16.	Clot formation	I.	Arteriosclerosis
_____ 17.	Cerebral vascular accident	J.	Thrombus

▷ *If you had difficulty with this section, review pages 400-402.*

CIRCULATION OF BLOOD

Circle the correct answer.

18. The aorta carries blood out of the:
    A. Right atrium
    B. Left atrium
    C. Right ventricle
    D. Left ventricle
    E. None of the above

19. The superior vena cava returns blood to the:
    A. Left atrium
    B. Left ventricle
    C. Right atrium
    D. Right ventricle
    E. None of the above

20. The _____ function as exchange vessels.
    A. Venules
    B. Capillaries
    C. Arteries
    D. Arterioles
    E. Veins

21. Blood returns from the lungs during pulmonary circulation via the:
    A. Pulmonary artery
    B. Pulmonary veins
    C. Aorta
    D. Inferior vena cava

22. The hepatic portal circulation serves the body by:
    A. Removing excess glucose and storing it in the liver as glycogen
    B. Detoxifying blood
    C. Assisting the body to maintain proper blood glucose balance
    D. All of the above

23. The structure used to bypass the liver in the fetal circulation is the:
    A. Foramen ovale
    B. Ductus venosus
    C. Ductus arteriosus
    D. Umbilical vein

24. The foramen ovale serves the fetal circulation by:
    A. Connecting the aorta and the pulmonary artery
    B. Shunting blood from the right atrium directly into the left atrium
    C. Bypassing the liver
    D. Bypassing the lungs

25. The structure used to connect the aorta and pulmonary artery in the fetal circulation is the:
    A. Ductus arteriosus
    B. Ductus venosus
    C. Aorta
    D. Foramen ovale

26. Which of the following is *not* an artery?
    A. Femoral
    B. Popliteal
    C. Coronary
    D. Inferior vena cava

 If you had difficulty with this section, review pages 402-406.

BLOOD PRESSURE
PULSE

If the statement is true, write "T" in the answer blank. If the statement is false, correct the statement by cir-
cling the incorrect term and writing the correct term in the answer blank.

_____ 27. Blood pressure is highest in the veins and lowest in the arteries.

_____ 28. The difference between two blood pressures is referred to as *blood pressure deficit*.

_____ 29. If the blood pressure in the arteries were to decrease so that it became equal to the average pressure in the arterioles, circulation would increase.

_____ 30. A stroke is often the result of low blood pressure.

_____ 31. Massive hemorrhage increases blood pressure.

_____ 32. Blood pressure is the volume of blood in the vessels.

_____ 33. Both the strength and the rate of heartbeat affect cardiac output and blood pressure.

_____ 34. The diameter of the arterioles helps determine how much blood drains out of arteries into arterioles.

_____ 35. A stronger heartbeat tends to decrease blood pressure and a weaker heartbeat tends to increase it.

_____ 36. The systolic pressure is the pressure being exerted against the vessels while the ventricles relax.

_____ 37. If blood becomes less viscous than normal, blood pressure increases.

_____ 38. A device called a *sphygmomanometer* is used to measure blood pressures in clinical situations.

_____ 39. Loud, tapping Korotkoff sounds suddenly begin when the cuff pressure measured by the mercury column equals the systolic pressure.

_____ 40. The venous blood pressure within the left atrium is called the *central venous pressure*.

_____ 41. The pulse is a vein expanding and then recoiling.

_____ 42. The radial artery is located at the wrist.

_____ 43. The common carotid artery is located in the neck along the front edge of the sternocleidomastoid muscle.

_____ 44. The artery located at the bend of the elbow that is used for locating the pulse is the dorsalis pedis.

 If you had difficulty with this section, review pages 406-413.

CIRCULATORY SHOCK

Fill in the blanks.

45. Complications of septicemia may result in _____
_____.

46. _____ _____ results from any type of heart failure.

47. An acute type of allergic reaction called _____ results in
_____ _____.

48. _____ _____ results from widespread dilation of blood vessels caused by an imbalance in autonomic stimulation of smooth muscles in vessel walls.

49. *Hypovolemia* means "_____ _____
_____."

50. A type of septic shock that results from staphylococcal infections that begin in the vagina of menstruating women and spread to the blood is _____
_____ _____.

▷ *If you had difficulty with this section, review pages 413-415.*

UNSCRAMBLE THE WORDS

51. **STMESYCI**

52. **NULVEE**

53. **RYTREA**

54. **USLEP**

Take the circled letters, unscramble them, and fill in the solution.

How Noah survived the flood.

55.

APPLYING WHAT YOU KNOW

56. Caryl was enjoying a picnic lunch one day when a bee suddenly flew down and stung her. Within seconds, Caryl began to experience difficulty breathing, tachycardia, a decrease in blood pressure, and cyanosis. What is Caryl experiencing?

57. Wilson was scheduled to undergo extensive surgery. His surgeon, Dr. Berger, requested that two units of blood be available for Wilson should he require them. What complication of surgery was Dr. Berger hoping to avoid?

58. Rochelle is a hairstylist who works long hours. Lately she has noticed that her feet are sore and edematous. What might be the cause of these symptoms? What advice could offer Rochelle some relief from these symptoms?

59. Rubin returned from surgery in stable condition. The nurse noted that each time she took Rubin's pulse and blood pressure, the pulse became higher and the blood pressure lower than the last time. What might be the cause?

60. Word Find

Find and circle 15 terms presented in this chapter. Words may be spelled top to bottom, bottom to top, right to left, left to right, or diagonally.

```
Y  H  Y  S  I  S  O  B  M  O  R  H  T  A  R
L  A  C  I  L  I  B  M  U  O  A  Y  N  I  Y
E  E  S  Y  S  T  E  M  I  C  C  G  D  E  U
M  V  E  N  U  L  E  D  D  C  I  X  M  D  I
E  Y  M  U  I  R  T  A  R  N  L  E  C  G  Y
N  O  I  T  A  Z  I  R  A  L  O  P  E  D  N
U  D  L  A  T  R  O  P  C  I  T  A  P  E  H
S  I  U  K  M  U  E  T  O  E  S  L  U  P  U
R  P  N  F  Y  C  B  E  D  R  A  L  Z  P  J
D  S  A  H  T  I  T  V  N  L  I  I  B  D  W
Q  U  R  O  I  V  A  Q  E  O  D  A  K  R  K
K  C  R  M  P  G  A  I  G  N  D  D  Z  Y  J
Y  I  Y  R  I  N  E  A  F  Z  L  Q  S  P  X
S  R  M  I  C  C  Q  O  A  W  U  N  H  O  K
P  T  A  V  H  H  Z  L  H  I  J  J  X  K  Z
```

Angina pectoris	ECG	Systemic
Apex	Endocardium	Thrombosis
Atrium	Hepatic portal	Tricuspid
Depolarization	Pulse	Umbilical
Diastolic	Semilunar	Venule

DID YOU KNOW?

Every pound of excess fat contains 200 miles of additional capillaries.

If laid out in a straight line, the average adult's circulatory system would be nearly 60,000 miles long—enough to circle the earth 2.5 times!

CIRCULATION OF THE BLOOD

Fill in the crossword puzzle.

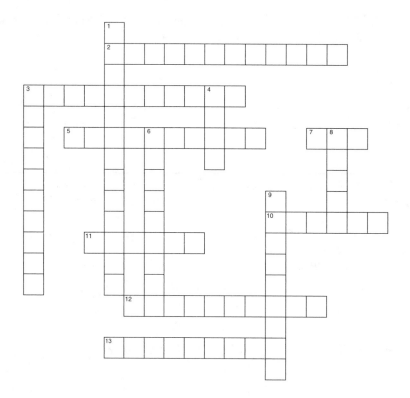

ACROSS

2. Inflammation of the lining of the heart
3. Bicuspid valve (two words)
5. Inner layer of pericardium
7. Cardiopulmonary resuscitation (abbreviation)
10. Carries blood away from the heart
11. Upper chamber of heart
12. Lower chambers of the heart
13. SA node

DOWN

1. Unique blood circulation through the liver (two words)
3. Muscular layer of the heart
4. Carries blood to the heart
6. Tiny artery
8. Heart rate
9. Carries blood from arterioles into venules

CHECK YOUR KNOWLEDGE

Multiple Choice

Circle the correct answer.

1. The medical term for high blood pressure is:
   A. Arteriosclerosis
   B. Cyanosis
   C. Hypertension
   D. Central venous pressure

2. Septic shock is caused by:
   A. Complications of toxins in the blood
   B. A nerve condition
   C. A drop in blood pressure
   D. Blood vessel dilation

3. Hypovolemic shock is caused by:
   A. Heart failure
   B. Dilated blood vessels
   C. A drop in blood volume
   D. A severe allergic reaction

4. Which vessels collect blood from the capillaries and return it to the heart?
   A. Arteries
   B. Sinuses
   C. Veins
   D. Arterioles

5. The innermost coat of an artery that comes into direct contact with blood is called the:
   A. Lumen
   B. Tunica externa
   C. Tunica intima
   D. Tunica media

6. Hemorrhoids can best be described as:
   A. Varicose veins
   B. Varicose veins in the rectum
   C. Thrombophlebitis of the rectum
   D. Clot formation in the rectum

7. In the fetal circulation:
   A. The ductus venosus allows most blood from the placenta to bypass the fetal liver.
   B. The umbilical vein carries oxygen-poor blood.
   C. The foramen ovale connects the aorta and the pulmonary artery.
   D. None of the above are true.

8. Which of the following events, if any, would *not* cause the blood pressure to increase?
   A. Hemorrhaging
   B. Increasing the viscosity of the blood
   C. Increasing the strength of the heartbeat
   D. All of the above

9. Arteriosclerosis is a disorder of the:
   A. Heart
   B. Veins
   C. Capillaries
   D. Arteries

10. A common type of vascular disease that occludes arteries by lipids and other matter is:
    A. Arteriosclerotic plaque
    B. Atherosclerosis
    C. Varicose veins
    D. Thrombophlebitis

Matching

Match each description in column A with its corresponding term in column B. (There is only one correct answer for each item.)

Column A

_____ 11. Largest artery
_____ 12. Decreased blood supply
_____ 13. Leg vein
_____ 14. Fetal circulation
_____ 15. Arterial procedure
_____ 16. Vein inflammation
_____ 17. Lung circulation
_____ 18. Weakened artery
_____ 19. Largest vein
_____ 20. Myocardial infarction

Column B

A.   Ischemia
B.   Phlebitis
C.   Foramen ovale
D.   Aneurysm
E.   Vena cava
F.   Angioplasty
G.   Aorta
H.   Pulmonary
I.   Great saphenous vein
J.   Cardiogenic shock

FETAL CIRCULATION

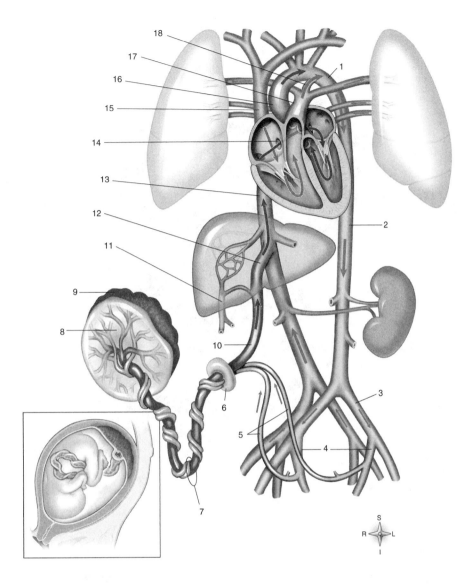

1. _____
2. _____
3. _____
4. _____
5. _____
6. _____
7. _____
8. _____
9. _____

10. _____
11. _____
12. _____
13. _____
14. _____
15. _____
16. _____
17. _____
18. _____

HEPATIC PORTAL CIRCULATION

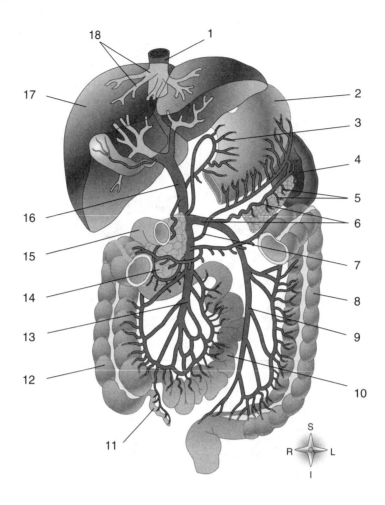

1. _____

2. _____

3. _____

4. _____

5. _____

6. _____

7. _____

8. _____

9. _____

10. _____

11. _____

12. _____

13. _____

14. _____

15. _____

16. _____

17. _____

18. _____

PRINCIPAL ARTERIES OF THE BODY

1. _____

2. _____

3. _____

4. _____

5. _____

6. _____

7. _____

8. _____

9. _____

10. _____

11. _____

12. _____

13. _____

14. _____

15. _____

16. _____

17. _____

18. _____

19. _____

20. _____

21. _____

22. _____

23. _____

24. _____

25. _____

26. _____

27. _____

28. _____

29. _____

30. _____

PRINCIPAL VEINS OF THE BODY

1. _____
2. _____
3. _____
4. _____
5. _____
6. _____
7. _____
8. _____
9. _____
10. _____
11. _____
12. _____
13. _____
14. _____
15. _____
16. _____
17. _____
18. _____
19. _____
20. _____
21. _____
22. _____
23. _____
24. _____
25. _____
26. _____
27. _____
28. _____
29. _____
30. _____
31. _____
32. _____
33. _____
34. _____
35. _____
36. _____
37. _____
38. _____

The Lymphatic System and Immunity

T he lymphatic system is similar to the circulatory system. Lymph, like blood, flows through an elaborate route of vessels. In addition to lymphatic vessels, the lymphatic system consists of lymph nodes, lymph, the thymus, tonsils, and the spleen. Unlike the circulatory system, the lymphatic vessels do not form a closed circuit. Lymph flows only once through the vessels before draining into the general blood circulation. This system is a filtering mechanism for microorganisms and serves as a protective device against foreign invaders such as cancer.

The immune system is the armed forces division of the body. Ready to attack at a moment's notice, the immune system defends us against the major enemies of the body: microorganisms, foreign transplanted tissue cells, and our own cells that have turned malignant.

The most numerous cells of the immune system are the lymphocytes. These cells circulate in the body's fluids seeking invading organisms and destroying them with powerful lymphotoxins, lymphokines, or antibodies.

Phagocytes, another large group of immune system cells, assist with the destruction of foreign invaders by a process known as *phagocytosis*. Neutrophils, monocytes, and connective tissue cells called *macrophages* use this process to surround unwanted microorganisms and ingest and digest them, rendering them harmless to the body.

Another weapon that the immune system possesses is complement. Normally a group of inactive enzymes present in the blood, complement can be activated to kill invading cells by drilling holes in their cytoplasmic membranes, which allows fluid to enter the cell until it bursts.

Your review of this chapter will give you an understanding of how the body defends itself from the daily invasion of destructive substances.

TOPICS FOR REVIEW

Before progressing to Chapter 16, you should familiarize yourself with the functions of the lymphatic system, the immune system, and the major structures that make up these systems. Your review should include knowledge of lymphatic vessels, lymph nodes, lymph, lymphatic organs and tissues, antibodies, complement, and the development of B and T cells. Your study should also include the differences in humoral and cell-mediated immunity. Finally, an understanding of the excessive responses of the immune system and immune system deficiencies are necessary to complete your review of this chapter.

THE LYMPHATIC SYSTEM

Fill in the blanks.

1. _____ *lymph* _____ is a specialized fluid formed in the tissue spaces that will be transported by way of specialized vessels to eventually reenter the circulatory system.

2. Blood plasma that has filtered out of capillaries into microscopic spaces between cells is called _____ *interstitial* _____ *fluid* _____.

3. Tiny blind-ended tubes distributed in the tissue spaces are called _____ *cisterna* _____ *chyli* _____.

4. Lymph eventually empties into two terminal vessels called the _____ _____ and the _____ _____.

5. The thoracic duct has an enlarged pouchlike structure called the _____ *cisterna* _____ *chyli* _____.

6. Lymph is filtered by moving through _____ *lymph* _____ *nodes* _____, which are located in clusters along the pathway of lymphatic vessels.

7. Lymph enters the node through four _____ *afferent* _____ lymph vessels.

8. Lymph exits the node through a single _____ *efferent* _____ lymph vessel.

9. An abnormal condition in which tissues exhibit edema because of the accumulation of lymph is _____ *lymphedema* _____.

10. Hodgkin disease is an example of _____.

▶ *If you had difficulty with this section, review pages 421-427.*

THYMUS
TONSILS
SPLEEN

Match each numbered description to one of the lymphatic system structures. Write the corresponding letter in the answer blank.

A. Thymus   B. Tonsils   C. Spleen

_____ 11. Palatine, pharyngeal, and lingual are examples

_____ 12. The largest lymphoid organ in the body

_____ 13. Destroys worn-out red blood cells

_____ 14. Located in the mediastinum

_____ 15. Serves as a reservoir for blood

_____ 16. T-lymphocytes

_____ 17. Largest at puberty

▶ *If you had difficulty with this section, review pages 427-428.*

THE IMMUNE SYSTEM

Match each term on the left with its corresponding description on the right.

_____ 18.	Nonspecific immunity	A.	Innate immunity
_____ 19.	Phagocytes	B.	Acquired immunity
_____ 20.	Specific immunity	C.	General protection
_____ 21.	Lymphocytes	D.	Artificial exposure
_____ 22.	Immunization	E.	Memory

IMMUNE SYSTEM MOLECULES

Match each description with its related term. Write the corresponding letter in the answer blank.

_____ 23.	A type of very specific antibodies produced from a population of identical cells	A.	Antibodies
_____ 24.	Protein compounds normally present in the body	B.	Antigen
_____ 25.	Also known as *antibody-mediated immunity*	C.	Monoclonal
_____ 26.	Combines with antibody to produce humoral immunity	D.	Complement cascade
_____ 27.	Antibody	E.	Complement
_____ 28.	The process of changing antibody molecule shape slightly to expose binding sites	F.	Humoral
_____ 29.	Capable of producing large quantities of very specific antibodies	G.	Combining site
_____ 30.	Inactive proteins in blood	H.	Hybridomas

▶ *If you had difficulty with this section, review pages 428-433.*

IMMUNE SYSTEM CELLS

Circle the correct answer.

31. The most numerous cells of the immune system are the:
    A. Monocytes
    B. Eosinophils
    C. Neutrophils
    D. Lymphocytes
    E. Complement

32. The second stage of B cell development changes a mature inactive B cell into a/an:
    A. Plasma cell
    B. Stem cell
    C. Antibody
    D. Activated B cell
    E. Immature B cell

33. Which one of the following is activated last in the immune process?
    A. Plasma cells
    B. Stem cells
    C. Antibodies
    D. Activated B cells
    E. Immature B cells

34. Which one of the following is part of the cell membrane of B cells?
    A. Complement
    B. Antigens
    C. Antibodies
    D. Epitopes
    E. None of the above

35. Immature B cells have:
    A. Four types of defense mechanisms on their cell membrane
    B. Several kinds of defense mechanisms on their cell membrane
    C. One specific kind of defense mechanism on their cell membrane
    D. No defense mechanisms on their cell membrane

36. Development of an active B cell depends on the B cell coming in contact with:
    A. Complement
    B. Antibodies
    C. Lymphotoxins
    D. Lymphokines
    E. Antigens

37. The kind of cell that produces large numbers of antibodies is the:
    A. B cell
    B. Stem cell
    C. T cell
    D. Memory cell
    E. Plasma cell

38. Just one of these short-lived cells that make antibodies can produce _____ of them per second.
    A. 20
    B. 200
    C. 2,000
    D. 20,000

39. Which of the following statements is *not* true of memory cells?
    A. They can secrete antibodies.
    B. They are found in lymph nodes.
    C. They develop into plasma cells.
    D. They can react with antigens.
    E. All of the above are true of memory cells.

40. T cell development begins in the:
    A. Lymph nodes
    B. Liver
    C. Pancreas
    D. Spleen
    E. Thymus

41. B cells function indirectly to produce:
    A. Humoral immunity
    B. Cell-mediated immunity
    C. Lymphotoxins
    D. Lymphokines

42. T cells function to produce:
    A. Humoral immunity
    B. Cell-mediated immunity
    C. Antibodies
    D. Memory cells

▷ *If you had difficulty with this section, review pages 433-438.*

HYPERSENSITIVITY OF THE IMMUNE SYSTEM

Circle the correct answer.

43. The term *allergy* is used to describe (*hypersensitivity* or *hyposensitivity*) of the immune system to relatively harmless environmental antigens.

44. Antigens that trigger an allergic response are often called (*antibodies* or *allergens*).

45. (*Anaphylactic shock* or *Urticaria*) is a life-threatening condition.

46. A common autoimmune disease is (*lupus* or *SCID*).

47. Erythroblastosis fetalis is an example of (*isoimmunity* or *autoimmunity*).

48. The antigens most commonly involved in transplant rejection are called (*SCIDs* or *HLAs*).

▷ *If you had difficulty with this section, review 438-441.*

IMMUNE DEFICIENCY

Match each condition with its origin. Write the corresponding letter in the answer blank.

A. Congenital   B.   Acquired (after birth)

_____ 49. AIDS

_____ 50. SCID

_____ 51. Improper B cell development

_____ 52. Viral infection

_____ 53. Genetic defect

▶ *If you had difficulty with this section, review pages 441-442.*

UNSCRAMBLE THE WORDS

54. **N T C M P E O L E M**

☐ ☐ ◯ ☐ ◯ ☐ ◯ ☐ ☐

55. **M T M Y I U N I**

☐ ◯ ☐ ☐ ☐ ☐ ☐ ☐

56. **O E N C L S**

◯ ◯ ☐ ☐ ◯ ☐

57. **F N R O E R T E N I**

☐ ☐ ☐ ☐ ◯ ☐ ◯ ☐ ◯

Take the circled letters, unscramble them, and fill in the solution.

What the student was praying for the night before exams.

58. ☐ ☐ ☐ ☐ ☐ ☐ ☐   ☐ ☐ ☐ ☐ ☐ ☐

...and please, don't let me forget to remember!

APPLYING WHAT YOU KNOW

59. Two-year old baby Metcalfe was exposed to chickenpox and subsequently developed the disease. What type of immunity will be developed as a result of this?

60. Marcia was a bisexual and an intravenous drug user. She has developed a type of skin cancer known as Kaposi sarcoma. What is Marcia's primary diagnosis?

61. Baby Wilson was born without a thymus gland. Immediate plans were made for a transplant to be performed. In the meantime, baby Wilson was placed in strict isolation. For what reason was he placed in isolation?

62. Word Find

Find and circle 14 terms presented in this chapter. Words may be spelled top to bottom, bottom to top, right to left, left to right, or diagonally.

```
I  N  F  L  A  M  M  A  T  O  R  Y  F  C  G
Q  N  L  O  Y  Z  O  C  C  P  A  O  F  S  X
M  W  T  A  A  M  N  J  X  Q  K  R  N  P  H
U  R  L  E  R  M  P  X  B  R  U  I  A  L  C
C  M  A  C  R  O  P  H  A  G  E  I  E  D  Z
X  M  N  D  K  F  M  N  O  T  U  C  R  N  M
A  E  O  R  E  Z  E  U  O  C  F  B  Y  E  B
Y  P  L  E  B  G  G  R  H  T  Y  T  S  E  D
Y  S  C  R  I  S  P  J  O  E  I  T  M  L  A
Z  M  O  T  J  X  E  T  O  N  A  E  E  P  X
T  O  N  S  I  L  S  S  U  M  Y  H  T  S  Y
W  A  O  C  J  N  I  M  W  K  O  Z  E  N  D
D  W  M  K  W  R  M  O  I  P  S  H  Y  B  G
F  H  W  U  J  I  Z  F  V  D  Z  L  Y  T  X
```

Acquired	Interferon	Proteins
Antigen	Lymph	Spleen
Humoral	Lymphocytes	Thymus
Immunity	Macrophage	Tonsils
Inflammatory	Monoclonal	

DID YOU KNOW?

In the United States, the HIV infection rate is increasing four times faster in women than in men. Women tend to underestimate their risk.

Ten percent of all HIV/AIDS cases are individuals 50 years of age and older.

LYMPH AND IMMUNITY

Fill in the crossword puzzle.

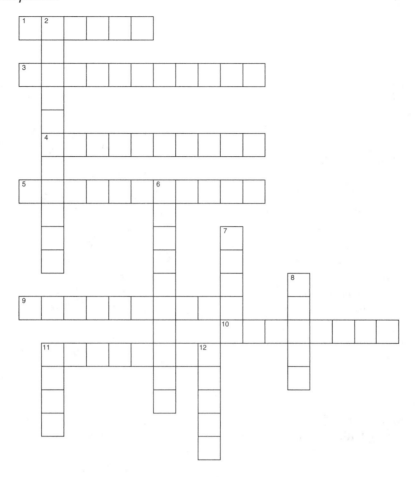

ACROSS

1. Largest lymphoid organ in the body
3. Connective tissue cells that are phagocytes
4. Protein compounds normally present in the body
5. Remain in reserve then turn into plasma cells when needed (two words)
9. Synthetically produced to fight certain diseases
10. Lymph exits the node through this lymph vessel
11. Lymph enters the node through these lymph vessels

DOWN

2. Secretes a copious amount of antibodies into the blood (two words)
6. Inactive proteins
7. Family of identical cells descended from one cell
8. Type of lymphocyte (humoral immunity—two words)
11. Immune deficiency disorder
12. Type of lymphocyte (cell-mediated immunity—two words)

CHECK YOUR KNOWLEDGE

Multiple Choice

Circle the correct answer.

1. T cells do which of the following?
   A. Develop in the thymus
   B. Form memory cells
   C. Form plasma cells
   D. All of the above

2. Lymph does which of the following?
   A. Forms as blood plasma filters out of capillaries
   B. Empties into the heart
   C. Flows through lymphatic arteries
   D. All of the above

3. Acquired immune deficiency syndrome is characterized by which of the following?
   A. Caused by a retrovirus
   B. Causes inadequate T cell formation
   C. Can result in death from cancer or infection
   D. All of the above

4. Interferon is:
   A. Produced by B cells
   B. A protein compound that protects other cells by interfering with the ability of a virus to reproduce
   C. A group of inactive enzyme proteins normally present in blood
   D. All of the above

5. B cells do which of the following?
   A. Develop into plasma cells and memory cells
   B. Establish humoral immunity
   C. Develop from primitive cells in bone marrow called *stem cells*
   D. All of the above

6. Which of the following functions to kill invading cells by drilling a hole in the plasma membrane?
   A. Interferon
   B. Complement cascade
   C. Antibody
   D. Memory cell

7. Which of the following cell types function in the immune system?
   A. Macrophages
   B. Lymphocytes
   C. T cells
   D. All of the above

8. Which of the following is an example of phagocytes?
   A. Dendritic cells
   B. Neutrophils
   C. Macrophages
   D. All of the above

9. What is a rapidly growing population of identical cells that produce large quantities of specific antibodies called?
   A. Complementary
   B. Lymphotoxic
   C. Chemotactic
   D. Monoclonal

10. Which of the following is a form of passive natural immunity?
    A. A child develops measles and acquires an immunity to subsequent infection.
    B. Antibodies are injected into an infected individual.
    C. An infant receives protection through its mother's milk.
    D. Vaccinations are given against smallpox.

Matching

Match each of the terms in column A with its corresponding description in column B. (Only one answer is correct for each.)

Column A

_____ 11. Adenoids

_____ 12. B cell

_____ 13. Clone

_____ 14. HIV virus

_____ 15. Complement

_____ 16. Filtration

_____ 17. Cisterna chyli

_____ 18. T cell

_____ 19. Vaccination

_____ 20. Antigen

Column B

A. Thoracic duct

B. Lymph node

C. Artificial immunity

D. Humoral immunity

E. Pharyngeal tonsils

F. Shaped to combine with an antibody

G. Inactive proteins

H. AIDS

I. Identical cells

J. Cell-mediated immunity

PRINCIPAL ORGANS OF THE LYMPHATIC SYSTEM

1. _____

2. _____

3. _____

4. _____

5. _____

6. _____

7. _____

8. _____

9. _____

10. _____

11. _____

12. _____

13. _____

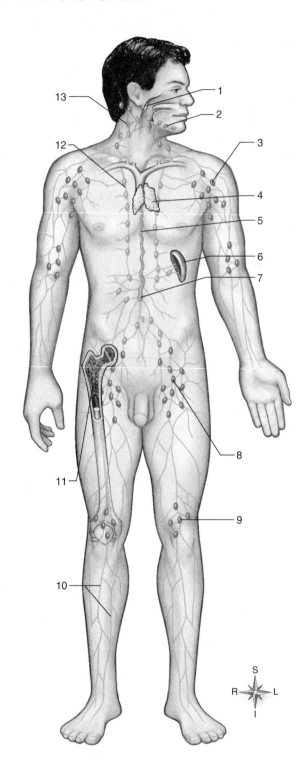

The Respiratory System

A s you sit reviewing this system, your body needs 16 quarts of air per minute. Walking requires 24 quarts of air, and running requires 50 quarts per minute. The respiratory system provides the air necessary for you to perform your daily activities and eliminates the waste gases from the air that you breathe. Take a deep breath, and think of the air as entering some 250 million tiny air sacs similar in appearance to clusters of grapes. These microscopic air sacs expand to let air in and contract to force it out. These tiny sacs, or alveoli, are the functioning units of the respiratory system. They provide the necessary volume of oxygen and eliminate carbon dioxide 24 hours a day.

Air enters either through the mouth or the nasal cavity. It next passes through the pharynx and past the epiglottis, through the glottis and the rest of the larynx. It then continues down the trachea, into the bronchi to the bronchioles, and finally through the alveoli. The reverse occurs for expelled air.

The exchange of gases between air in the lungs and in the blood is known as *external respiration*. The exchange of gases that occurs between the blood and the cells of the body is known as *internal respiration*. By constantly supplying adequate oxygen and removing carbon dioxide as it forms, the respiratory system helps maintain an environment conducive to maximum cell efficiency.

Your review of this system is necessary to provide you with an understanding of this essential homeostatic mechanism that supplies oxygen to our cells.

TOPICS FOR REVIEW

Before progressing to Chapter 17, you should have an understanding of the structure and function of the organs of the respiratory system. Your review should include knowledge of the mechanisms responsible for both internal and external respiration. Your study should conclude with a knowledge of the volumes of air exchanged in pulmonary ventilation, an understanding of how respiration is regulated, and the common disorders of the respiratory tract.

STRUCTURAL PLAN
RESPIRATORY TRACTS
RESPIRATORY MUCOSA

Match each term with its definition. Write the corresponding letter in the answer blank.

___J___ 1. Function of respiratory system
___G___ 2. Pharynx
___A___ 3. Passive transport process responsible for actual exchange of gases
___I___ 4. Assists with the movement of mucus toward the pharynx
___B___ 5. Barrier between the blood in the capillaries and the air in the alveolus
___F___ 6. Lines the tubes of the respiratory tree
___C___ 7. Terminal air sacs
___H___ 8. Trachea
___D___ 9. Surround alveoli
___E___ 10. Homeostatic mechanism

A. Diffusion
B. Respiratory membrane
C. Alveoli
D. Capillaries
E. Respiration
F. Respiratory mucosa
G. Upper respiratory tract
H. Lower respiratory tract
I. Cilia
J. Air distributor

Fill in the blanks.

The organs of the respiratory system are designed to perform two basic functions. They serve as an
(11) _____air_____ _____distributor_____ and as a
(12) _____gas_____ _____exchange_____. In addition to the
functions given above, the respiratory system (13) ___warms___,
(14) ___humidifies___, and (15) ___filters___ the air we
breathe. Respiratory organs include the (16) ___nose___,
(17) ___pharynx___, (18) ___larynx___,
(19) ___trachea___, (20) ___bronchi___, and the
(21) ___bronchioles lungs___. The respiratory system ends in millions of tiny, thin-walled sacs
called (22) ___alveolar ducts___. (23) ___alveoli diffusion___ of gases
takes place in these sacs. Two aspects of the structure of these sacs assist them in the exchange of gases. First,
an extremely thin membrane, the (24) ___respiratory___
___membrane___, allows for easy exchange, and second, the large number of air sacs
makes an enormous (25) ___surface___ area.

▷ *If you had difficulty with this section, review pages 453-457.*

NOSE
PHARYNX
LARYNX
DISORDERS OF UPPER RESPIRATORY TRACT

Circle the term in each word group that does not belong.

26. Nares   Septum   (Oropharynx)   Conchae

27. (Conchae)   Frontal   Maxillary   Sphenoidal

28. Oropharynx   (Throat)   5 inches   Epiglottis

29. Pharyngeal   Adenoids   Uvula   (Nasopharynx)

30. Middle ear   (Tubes)   Nasopharynx   Larynx

31. Voice box   Thyroid cartilage   Tonsils   Vocal cords

32. Palatine   Eustachian tube   Tonsils   (Oropharynx)

33. (Pharynx)   Epiglottis   Adam's apple   Voice box

Match each numbered term or phrase with the corresponding respiratory structure.

A. Nose   B. Pharynx   C. Larynx

___A___ 34. Warms and humidifies air

___B___ 35. Air and food pass through here

___A___ 36. Sinuses

___A___ 37. Conchae

___A___ 38. Septum

B ___C___ 39. Tonsils

B ___C___ 40. Middle ear infections

___C___ 41. Epiglottis

___A___ 42. Rhinitis

B ___C___ 43. Sore throat

___A___ 44. Epistaxis

▶ *If you had difficulty with this section, review pages 457-463.*

TRACHEA
BRONCHI, BRONCHIOLES, AND ALVEOLI
LUNGS AND PLEURA

Fill in the blanks.

45. The windpipe is more properly referred to as the ___trachea___ .

46. ___cartilage___ ensure that the framework of the trachea is almost noncollapsible.

47. A life-saving technique designed to free the trachea of ingested food or foreign objects is the ___heimlich___ ___maneuvor___ .

48. The first branch or division of the trachea leading to the lungs is the _____ _____ .

49. Each alveolar duct ends in several ___alveoli___ _____ .

50. The narrow part of each lung, up under the collarbone, is its _____ .

51. The ___parietal pleura___ covers the outer surface of the lungs and lines the inner surface of the rib cage.

52. Inflammation of the lining of the thoracic cavity is ___pleurisy___ .

53. The presence of air in the pleural space on one side of the chest is a ___pneumothorax___ .

▶ *If you had difficulty with this section, review pages 463-466.*

RESPIRATION

If the statement is true, write "T" in the answer blank. If the statement is false, correct the statement by circling the incorrect term and writing the correct term in the answer blank.

____F____ 54. Diffusion is the process that moves air into and out of the lungs.

____F____ 55. For inspiration to take place, the diaphragm and other respiratory muscles must relax.

____F____ 56. Diffusion is a passive process that results in movement up a concentration gradient.

____F____ 57. The exchange of gases that occurs between blood in tissue capillaries and the body cells is external respiration.

____T____ 58. Many different pulmonary volumes can be measured by having a person breathe into a spirometer.

____ 59. Ordinarily we take about 2 pints of air into our lungs with each breath.

____T____ 60. The amount of air normally breathed in and out with each breath is called *tidal volume.*

____F____ 61. The largest amount of air that one can breathe out in one expiration is called *residual volume.*

____T____ 62. The inspiratory reserve volume is the amount of air that can be forcibly inhaled after a normal inspiration.

▶ *If you had difficulty with this section, review pages 466-472.*

Circle the correct answer.

63. The term that means the same thing as breathing is:
    A. Gas exchange
    B. Respiration
    C. Inspiration
    D. Expiration
    E. Pulmonary ventilation

64. Carbaminohemoglobin is formed when _____ bind(s) to hemoglobin.
    A. Oxygen
    B. Amino acids
    C. Carbon dioxide
    D. Nitrogen
    E. None of the above

65. Most of the oxygen transported by the blood is:
    A. Dissolved into white blood cells
    B. Bound to white blood cells
    C. Bound to hemoglobin
    D. Bound to carbaminohemoglobin
    E. None of the above

66. Which of the following does *not* occur during inspiration?
    A. Elevation of the ribs
    B. Elevation of the diaphragm
    C. Contraction of the diaphragm
    D. Elongation of the chest cavity from top to bottom

67. A young adult male would have a vital capacity of about _____ mL.
    A. 500
    B. 1200
    C. 3300
    D. 4800
    E. 6200

68. The amount of air that can be forcibly exhaled after expiring the tidal volume is known as the:
    A. Total lung capacity
    B. Vital capacity
    C. Inspiratory reserve volume
    D. Expiratory reserve volume
    E. None of the above

69. Which one of the following formulas is correct?
    A. VC = TV - IRV + ERV
    B. VC = TV + IRV - ERV
    C. VC = TV + IRV × ERV
    D. VC = TV + IRV + ERV
    E. None of the above

▷ *If you had difficulty with this section, review pages 466-472.*

REGULATION OF RESPIRATION
RECEPTORS INFLUENCING RESPIRATION
TYPES OF BREATHING

Match each term on the left with the corresponding description on the right.

E	70.	Inspiratory center
B	71.	Chemoreceptors
G	72.	Pulmonary stretch receptors
A	73.	Dyspnea
F	74.	Respiratory arrest
D	75.	Eupnea
C	76.	Hypoventilation

A. Difficult breathing
B. Located in carotid bodies
C. Slow and shallow respirations
D. Normal respiratory rate
E. Located in the medulla
F. Failure to resume breathing after a period of apnea
G. Located throughout pulmonary airways and in the alveoli

 If you had difficulty with this section, review pages 472-474.

DISORDERS OF THE LOWER RESPIRATORY TRACT

Fill in the blanks.

77. _____*pneumonia*_____ is an acute inflammation of the lungs in which the alveoli and bronchi become plugged with thick fluid.

78. _____ is still a major cause of death in many poor, densely populated regions of the world. It has recently reemerged as an important health problem in some major U.S. cities.

79. _____*emphysema*_____ may result from the progression of chronic bronchitis or other conditions as air becomes trapped within alveoli, causing them to enlarge and eventually rupture.

80. _____*asthma*_____ is an obstructive disorder characterized by recurring spasms of the smooth muscle in the walls of the bronchial air passages.

▷ *If you had difficulty with this section, review pages 474-479.*

UNSCRAMBLE THE WORDS

81. **S P U E L I R Y**

P I E U R I S Y

82. **C R N B O S I T H I**

83. **S E S X P T I A I**

E P I T A

84. **D D N E A O I S**

Take the circled letters, unscramble them, and fill in the solution.

What Mona Lisa was to DaVinci.

85. ⬚⬚⬚⬚⬚⬚⬚⬚⬚⬚⬚⬚

APPLYING WHAT YOU KNOW

86. Mr. Gorski is a heavy smoker. Recently he has noticed that when he gets up in the morning, he has a bothersome cough that brings up a large accumulation of mucus. This cough persists for several minutes and then leaves until the next morning. What is an explanation for this problem?

87. Penny is 5 years old and is a mouth breather. She has had repeated episodes of tonsillitis, and her pediatrician, Dr. Smith, has suggested removal of her tonsils and adenoids. He further suggests that the surgery will probably cure her mouth breathing problem. Why is this a possibility?

88. Sandy developed emphysema. This disease reduces the capacity of the lungs to recoil elastically. Which respiratory air volumes will this condition affect? Why?

89. Word Find

Find and circle 14 terms presented in this chapter. Words may be spelled top to bottom, bottom to top, right to left, left to right, or diagonally.

```
N  K  S  A  Q  B  I  L  V  A  D  T  I  X  D
O  X  O  O  B  F  I  F  G  I  M  N  R  G  Y
I  G  N  X  W  D  E  E  F  L  B  A  U  T  S
T  B  K  Y  N  H  E  F  O  I  U  T  I  R  P
A  T  M  H  E  O  U  T  R  C  C  C  P  V  N
L  L  A  E  P  S  I  R  I  Z  A  A  N  F  E
I  P  T  M  I  H  G  T  I  P  R  F  P  C  A
T  U  B  O  G  Q  E  V  A  Q  O  R  V  N  W
N  L  N  G  L  R  J  C  C  R  T  U  P  D  C
E  M  U  L  O  V  L  A  U  D  I  S  E  R  E
V  O  V  O  T  A  N  G  J  E  D  P  Z  U  U
O  N  K  B  T  C  N  U  U  E  B  O  S  J  S
P  A  L  I  I  K  E  U  C  N  O  Z  K  N  A
Y  R  V  N  S  D  I  O  N  E  D  A  M  F  I
H  Y  O  M  L  O  A  Z  D  T  Y  M  N  L  K
```

Adenoids	Epiglottis	Residual volume
Carotid body	Hypoventilation	Surfactant
Cilia	Inspiration	URI
Diffusion	Oxyhemoglobin	Vital capacity
Dyspnea	Pulmonary	

DID YOU KNOW?

If the alveoli in our lungs were flattened out they would cover one-half of a tennis court.

Eighty percent of lung cancer cases are due to cigarette smoking.

RESPIRATORY SYSTEM

Fill in the crossword puzzle.

ACROSS

1. Device used to measure the amount of air exchanged in breathing
6. Expiratory reserve volume (abbreviation)
7. Sphenoidal (two words)
8. Terminal air sacs
9. Shelflike structures that protrude into the nasal cavity
11. Inflammation of pleura
12. Respirations stop

DOWN

2. Surgical procedure to remove tonsils
3. Doctor who developed life-saving technique
4. Windpipe
5. Trachea branches into right and left structures
10. Voice box

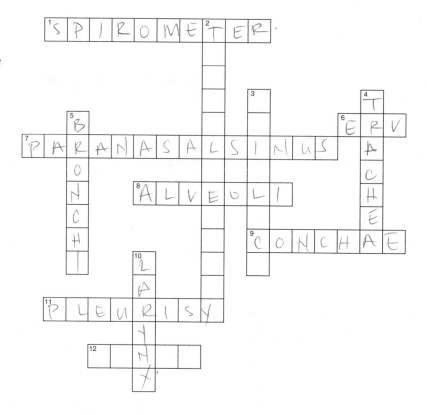

CHECK YOUR KNOWLEDGE

Multiple Choice

Circle the correct answer.

1. Chemoreceptors in the carotid and aortic bodies are characterized by which of the following?
   A. Sensitive to increases in blood carbon dioxide level
   B. Found in the brain
   C. Sensitive to increases in blood oxygen level
   D. Send impulses to the heart

2. What is the lowest segment of the pharynx called?
   A. Oropharynx
   B. Laryngopharynx
   C. Nasopharynx
   D. Hypopharynx

3. What is the narrow upper portion of a lung called?
   A. Base
   B. Notch
   C. Costal surface
   D. Apex

4. What is the largest amount of air that a person can breathe in and out in one inspiration and expiration called?
   A. Tidal volume
   B. Vital capacity
   C. Residual volume
   D. Inspiratory reserve volume

5. Which of the following statements, if any, is *not* characteristic of human lungs?
    A. Both right and left lungs are composed of three lobes.
    B. Bronchi subdivide to form bronchioles.
    C. Capillary supply is abundant to facilitate gas exchange.
    D. All of the above statements are characteristic of human lungs.

6. Which body function is made possible by the existence of fibrous bands stretched across the larynx?
    A. Swallowing
    B. Breathing
    C. Diffusion
    D. Speech

7. The trachea is almost noncollapsible because of the presence of which of the following?
    A. Rings of cartilage
    B. Thyroid cartilage
    C. Epiglottis
    D. Vocal cords

8. Which of the following is true of the exchange of respiratory gases between lungs and blood?
    A. It takes place by diffusion.
    B. It is called *external respiration*.
    C. Both A and B are true.
    D. None of the above is true.

9. When the diaphragm contracts, which phase of ventilation is taking place?
    A. External respiration
    B. Expiration
    C. Internal respiration
    D. Inspiration

10. Which of the following is *not* characteristic of the nasal cavities?
    A. They contain many blood vessels that warm incoming air.
    B. They contain the adenoids.
    C. They are lined with mucous membranes.
    D. They are separated by a partition called the *nasal septum*.

Matching

Match each term in column A with its corresponding term in column B. (Only one answer is correct for each.)

Column A

_____ 11. Vocal cords

_____ 12. Pulmonary ventilation

_____ 13. Pleura

_____ 14. Pneumothorax

_____ 15. Emphysema

_____ 16. Throat

_____ 17. Ethmoidal

_____ 18. Windpipe

_____ 19. Alveoli

_____ 20. Surfactant

Column B

A. Serous membrane

B. Pharynx

C. Paranasal sinus

D. LVRS

E. Larynx

F. Diffusion

G. Collapsed lung

H. Trachea

I. Breathing

J. IRDS

SAGITTAL VIEW OF FACE AND NECK

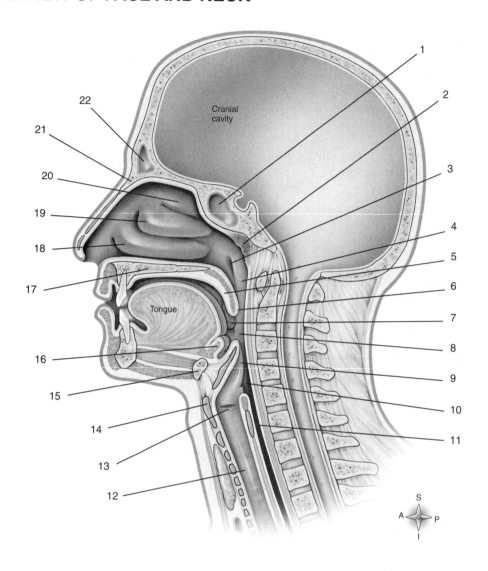

1. _____

2. _____

3. _____

4. _____

5. _____

6. _____

7. _____

8. _____

9. _____

10. _____

11. _____

12. _____

13. _____

14. _____

15. _____

16. _____

17. _____

18. _____

19. _____

20. _____

21. _____

22. _____

RESPIRATORY ORGANS

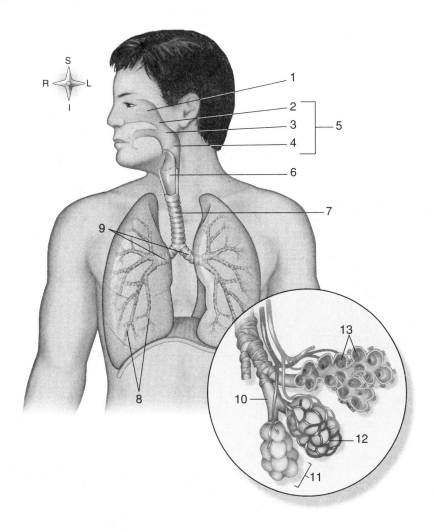

1. _____

2. _____

3. _____

4. _____

5. _____

6. _____

7. _____

8. _____

9. _____

10. _____

11. _____

12. _____

13. _____

PULMONARY VENTILATION VOLUMES

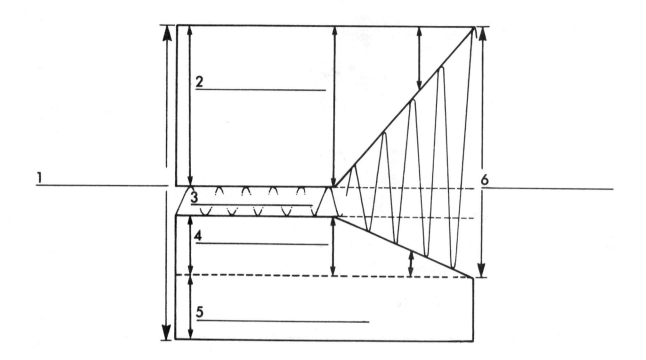

1. _____   4. _____

2. _____   5. _____

3. _____   6. _____

CHAPTER 17

The Digestive System

T hink of the last meal you ate. Imagine the different shapes, sizes, tastes, and textures that you so recently enjoyed. Think of those items circulating in your bloodstream in those same original shapes, sizes, and textures. Impossible? Of course! Because of this impossibility, you can begin to understand and marvel at the close relationship of the digestive system to the circulatory system. It is the digestive system that changes our food, both mechanically and chemically, into a form that is usable in the blood and the body.

This change in food begins the moment you take the very first bite. Digestion starts in the mouth, where food is chewed and mixed with saliva. It then moves down the pharynx and esophagus by peristalsis and enters the stomach. In the stomach it is churned and mixed with gastric juices to become chyme. The chyme goes from the stomach into the duodenum where it is further broken down chemically by intestinal fluids, bile, and pancreatic juice. Those secretions prepare the food for absorption all along the course of the small intestine. Products that are not absorbed pass on through the entire length of the small intestine (duodenum, jejunum, ileum). From there they enter into the cecum of the large intestine, continue on to the ascending colon, transverse colon, descending colon, and sigmoid colon, and finally into the rectum, and out the anus.

Products that are used in the cells undergo absorption. Absorption allows newly processed nutrients to pass through the walls of the digestive tract and into the bloodstream to be distributed to the cells.

Your review of this system will help you understand the mechanical and chemical processes necessary to convert food into energy sources and compounds necessary for survival.

TOPICS FOR REVIEW

Before progressing to Chapter 18, you should review the structure and function of all the organs of digestion. You should have an understanding of the process of digestion, both chemical and mechanical, and of the processes of absorption and metabolism.

THE DIGESTIVE SYSTEM
ORGANS OF THE DIGESTIVE SYSTEM

Fill in the blanks.

1. The organs of the digestive system form an irregular-shaped tube called the *alimentary canal* or

    _____ _____.

2. The churning of food in the stomach is an example of the _____ break-
    down of food.

3. _____ breakdown occurs when digestive enzymes act on food as it
    passes through the digestive tract.

4. Waste material resulting from the digestive process is known as _____.

5. Foods undergo three kinds of processing in the body: _____,
    _____, and _____.

Identify which are main organs and which are accessory organs of the digestive system. Write the corresponding letter in the answer blank.

A. Main organ   B. Accessory organ

_____ 6.   Mouth

_____ 7.   Parotids

_____ 8.   Liver

_____ 9.   Stomach

_____ 10.   Cecum

_____ 11.   Esophagus

_____ 12.   Rectum

_____ 13.   Pharynx

_____ 14.   Appendix

_____ 15.   Teeth

_____ 16.   Gallbladder

_____ 17.   Pancreas

▶ *If you had difficulty with this section, review pages 487-488.*

MOUTH

TEETH

SALIVARY GLANDS

Circle the correct answer.

18. Which one of the following is *not* a part of the roof of the mouth?
    A. Uvula
    B. Palatine bones
    C. Maxillary bones
    D. Soft palate
    E. All of the above are part of the roof of the mouth.

19. The largest of the papillae on the surface of the tongue are the:
    A. Filiform
    B. Fungiform
    C. Vallate
    D. Taste buds

20. The first baby tooth, on average, appears at:
    A. 2 months
    B. 1 year
    C. 3 months
    D. 1 month
    E. 6 months

21. The portion of the tooth that is covered with enamel is the:
    A. Pulp cavity
    B. Neck
    C. Root
    D. Crown
    E. None of the above is correct.

22. The wall of the pulp cavity is surrounded by:
    A. Enamel
    B. Dentin
    C. Cementum
    D. Connective tissue
    E. Blood and lymphatic vessels

23. Which of the following teeth is missing from the deciduous arch?
    A. Central incisor
    B. Canine
    C. Second premolar
    D. First molar
    E. Second molar

24. The permanent central incisor erupts between the ages of _____.
    A. 9 and 13
    B. 5 and 6
    C. 7 and 10
    D. 7 and 8
    E. None of the above

25. The third molar appears between the ages of _____.
    A. 10 and 14
    B. 5 and 8
    C. 11 and 16
    D. 17 and 24
    E. None of the above

26. A general term for infection of the gums is:
    A. Dental caries
    B. Leukoplakia
    C. Vincent angina
    D. Gingivitis

27. The ducts of the _____ glands open into the floor of the mouth.
    A. Sublingual
    B. Submandibular
    C. Parotid
    D. Carotid

28. The volume of saliva secreted per day is about:
    A. One-half pint
    B. One pint
    C. One liter
    D. One gallon

29. Mumps are an infection of the:
    A. Parotid gland
    B. Sublingual gland
    C. Submandibular gland
    D. Tonsils

30. Incisors are used during mastication to:
    A. Cut
    B. Piece
    C. Tear
    D. Grind

31. Another name for the third molar is:
    A. Central incisor
    B. Wisdom tooth
    C. Canine
    D. Lateral incisor

32. After food has been chewed, it is formed into a small rounded mass called a:
    A. Moat
    B. Chyme
    C. Bolus
    D. Protease

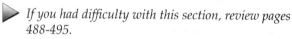 *If you had difficulty with this section, review pages 488-495.*

WALL OF DIGESTIVE TRACT

Fill in the blanks.

33. The serosa of the digestive tube is composed of the _____ _____ in the abdominal cavity.

34. The digestive tract extends from the _____ to the _____.

35. The inside or hollow space within the alimentary canal is called the _____.

36. The inside layer of the digestive tract is the _____.

37. The connective tissue layer that lies beneath the lining of the digestive tract is the _____.

38. The muscularis contracts and moves food through the gastrointestinal tract by a process known as _____.

39. The outermost covering of the digestive tube is the _____.

40. The loops of the digestive tract are anchored to the posterior wall of the abdominal cavity by the _____.

PHARYNX

ESOPHAGUS

STOMACH

Fill in the blanks.

The (41) _____ is a tubelike structure that functions as part of both the respiratory and digestive systems. It connects the mouth with the (42) _____. The esophagus serves as a passageway for movement of food from the pharynx to the (43) _____. Food enters the stomach by passing through the muscular (44) _____ _____ at the end of the esophagus. Contraction of the stomach mixes the food thoroughly with the gastric juices and breaks it down into a semisolid mixture called (45) _____. The three divisions of the stomach are the (46) _____, (47) _____, and (48) _____. Food is held in the stomach by the (49) _____ _____ muscle long enough for partial digestion to occur. After food has been in the stomach for approximately 3 hours, the chyme will enter the (50) _____ _____.

Match each term with its corresponding definition.

_____ 51. Stomach folds

_____ 52. Upper right border of stomach

_____ 53. Heartburn

_____ 54. 10-inch passageway

_____ 55. Shown to be an effective treatment of Crohn disease

_____ 56. Semisolid mixture of stomach contents

_____ 57. Muscle contractions of the digestive system

_____ 58. Craterlike wound in digestive system caused by tissue destruction

_____ 59. Stomach pushes through the gap in the diaphragm

_____ 60. Lower left border of stomach

A. Esophagus

B. Chyme

C. Peristalsis

D. Rugae

E. Ulcer

F. Greater curvature

G. Acid indigestion

H. Triple therapy

I. Hiatal hernia

J. Lesser curvature

▷ *If you had difficulty with this section, review pages 495-501.*

SMALL INTESTINE
LIVER AND GALLBLADDER
PANCREAS

Circle the correct answer.

61. Which one is *not* part of the small intestine?
    A. Jejunum
    B. Ileum
    C. Cecum
    D. Duodenum

62. Which one of the following structures does *not* increase the surface area of the intestine for absorption?
    A. Plicae
    B. Rugae
    C. Villi
    D. Brush border

63. The union of the cystic duct and hepatic duct form the:
    A. Common bile duct
    B. Major duodenal papilla
    C. Minor duodenal papilla
    D. Pancreatic duct

64. Obstruction of the _____ will lead to jaundice.
    A. Hepatic duct
    B. Pancreatic duct
    C. Cystic duct
    D. None of the above

65. Bile is responsible for the:
    A. Final digestion of fats
    B. Emulsification of fats
    C. Chemical breakdown of fats
    D. Chemical breakdown of cholesterol

66. The middle third of the duodenum contains the:
    A. Islets
    B. Fundus
    C. Body
    D. Rugae
    E. Major duodenal papilla

67. Cholelithiasis is the term used to describe:
    A. Biliary colic
    B. Jaundice
    C. Portal hypertension
    D. Gall stones

68. The liver is an:
    A. Enzyme
    B. Endocrine organ
    C. Endocrine gland
    D. Exocrine gland

69. Fats in chyme stimulate the secretion of the hormone:
    A. Lipase
    B. Cholecystokinin
    C. Protease
    D. Amylase

70. The largest gland in the body is the:
    A. Pituitary
    B. Thyroid
    C. Liver
    D. Thymus

 If you had difficulty with this section, review pages 501-508.

LARGE INTESTINE
APPENDIX
PERITONEUM

If the statement is true, write "T" in the answer blank. If the statement is false, correct the statement by circling the incorrect term and writing the correct term in the answer blank.

_____ 71. Bacteria in the large intestine are responsible for the synthesis of vitamin E needed for normal blood clotting.

_____ 72. Villi in the large intestine absorb salts and water.

_____ 73. If waste products pass rapidly through the large intestine, constipation results.

_____ 74. The ileocecal valve opens into the sigmoid colon.

_____ 75. The splenic flexure is the bend between the ascending colon and the transverse colon.

_____ 76. The splenic colon is the S-shaped segment that terminates in the rectum.

_____ 77. The appendix serves no important digestive function in humans.

_____ 78. Appendicitis is more common in children and young adults because the lumen of the appendix is larger during that period making it easier for food and fecal material to become trapped.

_____ 79. The visceral layer of the peritoneum lines the abdominal cavity.

_____ 80. The greater omentum is shaped like a fan and serves to anchor the small intestine to the posterior abdominal wall.

_____ 81. Diarrhea is an inflammation of abnormal saclike outpouchings of the intestinal wall.

_____ 82. Crohn disease is a type of autoimmune colitis.

_____ 83. A colostomy is a surgical procedure in which an artificial anus is created on the abdominal wall.

_____ 84. Peritonitis is the abnormal accumulation of fluid in the peritoneal space.

 If you had difficulty with this section, review pages 508-513.

DIGESTION

ABSORPTION

Circle the correct answer.

85. Which one of the following substances does *not* contain any enzymes?
   A. Saliva
   B. Bile
   C. Gastric juice
   D. Pancreatic juice
   E. Intestinal juice

86. Which one of the following is a simple sugar?
   A. Maltose
   B. Sucrose
   C. Lactose
   D. Glucose
   E. Starch

87. Cane sugar is the same as:
   A. Maltose
   B. Lactose
   C. Sucrose
   D. Glucose
   E. None of the above

88. Most of the digestion of carbohydrates takes place in the:
   A. Mouth
   B. Stomach
   C. Small intestine
   D. Large intestine

89. Fats are broken down into:
   A. Amino acids
   B. Simple sugars
   C. Fatty acids
   D. Disaccharides

 If you had difficulty with this section, review pages 513-516.

CHEMICAL DIGESTION

90. Fill in the blank areas on the chart below.

DIGESTIVE JUICES AND ENZYMES	SUBSTANCE DIGESTED (OR HYDROLYZED)	RESULTING PRODUCT
Saliva		
1. Amylase	1.	1. Maltose
Gastric Juice		
2. Protease (pepsin) plus hydrochloric acid	2. Proteins	2.
Pancreatic Juice		
3. Protease (trypsin)	3. Proteins (intact or partially digested)	3.
4. Lipase	4.	4. Fatty acids, monoglycerides, and glycerol
5. Amylase	5.	5. Maltose
Intestinal Juice		
6. Peptidases	6.	6. Amino acids
7.	7. Sucrose	7. Glucose and fructose
8. Lactase	8.	8. Glucose and galactose (simple sugars)
9. Maltase	9. Maltose	9.

▶ *If you had difficulty with this section, review page 515.*

UNSCRAMBLE THE WORDS

91. **S L B O U**

☐ ◯ ☐ ◯ ☐ ☐

92. **E Y C H M**

◯ ☐ ☐ ☐ ◯

93. **L L A A P P I**

☐ ◯ ☐ ☐ ☐ ☐ ◯

94. **P M E R T E U I O N**

◯ ☐ ◯ ☐ ☐ ☐ ◯ ☐ ☐ ☐

Take the circled letters, unscramble them, and fill in the solution.

What the groom gave his bride after the wedding.

95. ☐ ☐ ☐ ☐   ☐ ☐ ☐ ☐ ☐

APPLYING WHAT YOU KNOW

96. Mr. Amoto was a successful businessman, but he worked too hard and was always under great stress. He took high doses of aspirin, almost daily, to relieve his stress headaches. His doctor cautioned him that if he did not alter his style of living, he would be subject to hyperacidity. What could be a result of hyperacidity?

97. Baby Nicholas has been regurgitating his bottle feeding at every meal. The milk is curdled, but does not appear to be digested. He has become dehydrated, and so his mother, Bobbi, is taking him to the pediatrician. What would you guess is a possible diagnosis based on what you have learned from your textbook reading?

98. Mr. Lynch has high cholesterol. In an effort to lower his cholesterol, he quickly lost 25 pounds by consuming an ultra low-fat diet. Since then he has noticed a yellowish cast to his skin and has periodic pain in the right upper quadrant of the abdominopelvic region. What is a possible diagnosis for Mr. Lynch? What is the name of the surgical procedure that may be performed on Mr. Lynch?

99.   Word Find

Find and circle 22 terms presented in this chapter. Words may be spelled top to bottom, bottom to top, right to left, left to right, or diagonally.

```
X  M  E  T  A  B  O  L  I  S  M  X  X  W
R  S  D  P  E  R  I  S  T  A  L  S  I  S
E  V  A  M  N  O  I  T  S  E  G  I  D  R
E  D  E  E  U  O  Q  T  W  Q  O  H  N  Q
Q  Z  H  S  R  N  I  N  T  F  E  C  E  S
D  H  R  E  C  C  I  T  K  C  J  A  P  E
Q  W  R  N  A  T  N  V  P  Y  R  M  P  C
O  C  A  T  N  R  B  A  P  R  H  O  A  I
U  Y  I  E  O  W  T  A  P  A  O  T  W  D
B  O  D  R  L  N  P  B  F  Q  J  S  V  N
N  T  S  Y  F  I  S  L  U  M  E  E  B  U
W  G  J  A  L  U  V  U  N  R  N  W  O  A
Q  S  N  L  X  D  U  O  D  E  N  U  M  J
H  C  A  V  I  T  Y  M  U  C  O  S  A  D
Y  E  A  A  P  H  V  W  S  V  C  Q  J  C
```

Absorption	Emulsify	Mucosa
Appendix	Feces	Pancreas
Cavity	Fundus	Papillae
Crown	Heartburn	Peristalsis
Dentin	Jaundice	Stomach
Diarrhea	Mastication	Uvula
Digestion	Mesentery	
Duodenum	Metabolism	

DID YOU KNOW?

The liver performs over 500 functions and produces over 1000 enzymes to handle the chemical conversions necessary for survival.

About 20% of older adults have diabetes, and almost 40% have some impaired glucose tolerance.

The human stomach lining replaces itself every 3 days.

DIGESTIVE SYSTEM

Fill in the crossword puzzle.

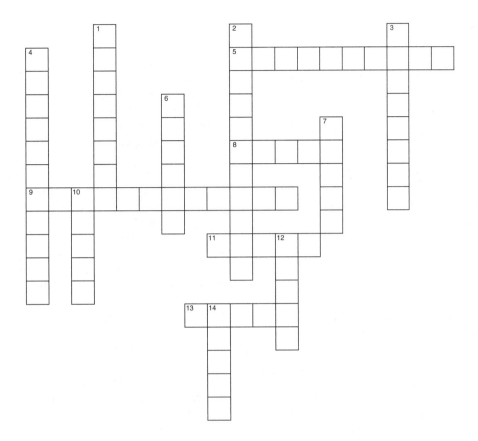

ACROSS

5. Digested food moves from intestine to blood
8. Semisolid mixture
9. Inflammation of the appendix
11. Rounded mass of food
13. Stomach folds

DOWN

1. Yellowish skin discoloration
2. Process of chewing
3. Fluid stools
4. Movement of food through digestive tract
6. Vomitus
7. Waste product of digestion
10. Intestinal folds
12. Open wound in digestive area acted on by acid juices
14. Prevents food from entering nasal cavities

CHECK YOUR KNOWLEDGE

Multiple Choice

Circle the correct answer.

1. During the process of digestion, *stored* bile is poured into the duodenum by which of the following?
   A. Gallbladder
   B. Liver
   C. Pancreas
   D. Spleen

2. Which portion of the alimentary canal mixes food with gastric juice and breaks it down into a mixture called *chyme*?
   A. Gallbladder
   B. Small intestine
   C. Stomach
   D. Large intestine

3. What is the middle portion of the small intestine called?
   A. Jejunum
   B. Ileum
   C. Duodenum
   D. Cecum

4. The crown of the tooth is covered externally with which of the following?
   A. Cementum
   B. Enamel
   C. Dentin
   D. Pulp

5. What is the layer of tissue that forms the outermost covering of organs found in the digestive tract called?
   A. Mucosa
   B. Serosa
   C. Submucosa
   D. Muscularis

6. Duodenal ulcers appear in which of the following?
   A. Stomach
   B. Small intestine
   C. Large intestine
   D. Esophagus

7. What is an extension of the peritoneum that is shaped like a giant pleated fan?
   A. Omentum
   B. Mesentery
   C. Peritoneal cavity
   D. Ligament

8. Protein digestion begins in the:
   A. Esophagus
   B. Small intestine
   C. Stomach
   D. Large intestine

9. The enzyme pepsin is concerned primarily with the digestion of which of the following?
   A. Sugars
   B. Starches
   C. Proteins
   D. Fats

10. The enzyme amylase converts which of the following?
    A. Starches to sugars
    B. Sugars to starches
    C. Proteins to amino acids
    D. Fatty acids and glycerol to fats

Completion

Fill in the blanks using the terms listed below. Write the corresponding letter in each blank.

A. Ileum	G. Lower esophageal sphincter	M. Upper esophageal sphincter	S. Premolars
B. Amylase	H. Digestion	N. Sigmoid colon	T. Mucosa
C. Muscularis	I. Incisors	O. Canines	U. Submucosa
D. Metabolism	J. Greater omentum	P. Amino acids	V. Cecum
E. Cholecystokinin	K. Absorption	Q. Duodenum	W. Bile
F. Molars	L. Adventitia	R. Jejunum	X. Serosa

11. The S-shaped portion of the colon is called the _____.

12. The portion of the peritoneum that descends from the stomach and the transverse colon to form a lacy apron of fat over the intestines is called the _____.

13. The "building blocks" of protein molecules are _____.

14. The small intestine is made up of three sections called the _____, _____, and the _____.

15. Fats that enter into the digestive tract are emulsified when they are acted on by a substance called _____.

16. Foods undergo three kinds of processing in the body: _____, _____, and _____.

17. Fats in the chyme stimulate the secretion of _____, which stimulates contraction of the gallbladder to release bile.

18. The four tissue layers that make up the wall of the digestive tract are the _____, _____, _____, and _____.

19. Food enters the stomach by passing through a muscular structure at the end of the esophagus. This structure is called the _____.

20. The four major types of teeth found in the human mouth are _____, _____, _____, and _____.

LOCATION OF DIGESTIVE ORGANS

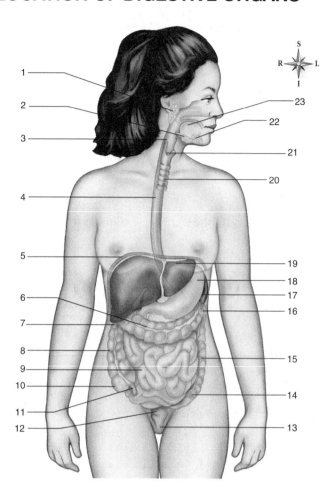

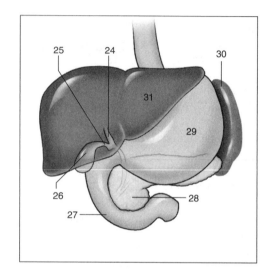

1. _____
2. _____
3. _____
4. _____
5. _____
6. _____
7. _____
8. _____
9. _____
10. _____
11. _____
12. _____
13. _____
14. _____
15. _____
16. _____

17. _____
18. _____
19. _____
20. _____
21. _____
22. _____
23. _____
24. _____
25. _____
26. _____
27. _____
28. _____
29. _____
30. _____
31. _____

TOOTH

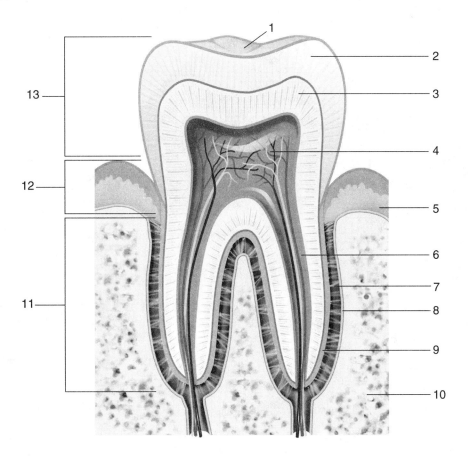

1. _____
2. _____
3. _____
4. _____
5. _____
6. _____
7. _____

8. _____
9. _____
10. _____
11. _____
12. _____
13. _____

THE SALIVARY GLANDS

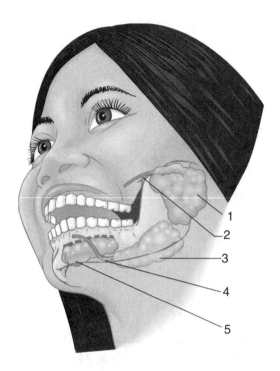

1. _____   4. _____

2. _____   5. _____

3. _____

STOMACH

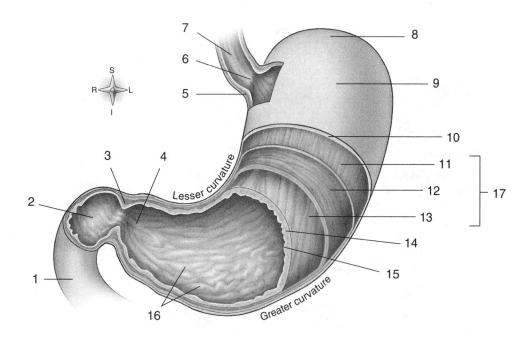

1. _____

2. _____

3. _____

4. _____

5. _____

6. _____

7. _____

8. _____

9. _____

10. _____

11. _____

12. _____

13. _____

14. _____

15. _____

16. _____

17. _____

GALLBLADDER AND BILE DUCTS

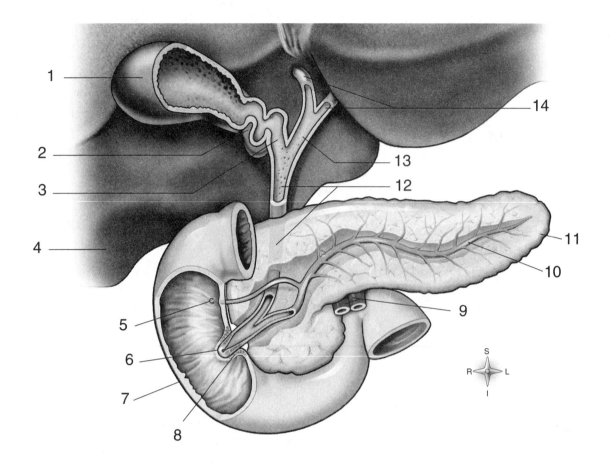

1. _____

2. _____

3. _____

4. _____

5. _____

6. _____

7. _____

8. _____

9. _____

10. _____

11. _____

12. _____

13. _____

14. _____

THE SMALL INTESTINE

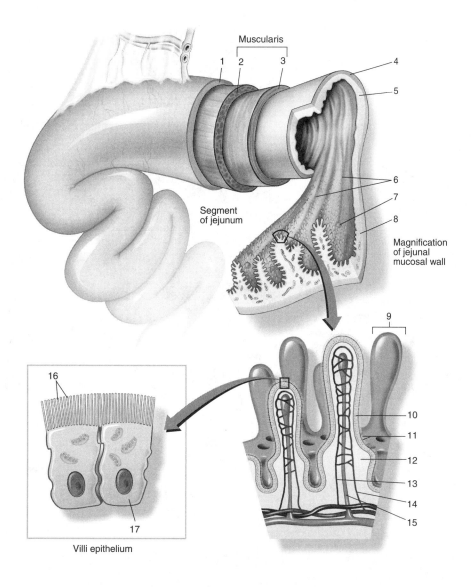

1. _____
2. _____
3. _____
4. _____
5. _____
6. _____
7. _____
8. _____
9. _____

10. _____
11. _____
12. _____
13. _____
14. _____
15. _____
16. _____
17. _____

THE LARGE INTESTINE

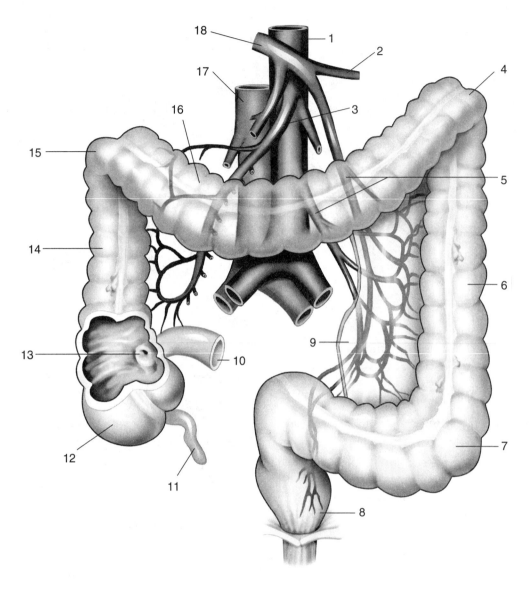

1. _____   10. _____

2. _____   11. _____

3. _____   12. _____

4. _____   13. _____

5. _____   14. _____

6. _____   15. _____

7. _____   16. _____

8. _____   17. _____

9. _____   18. _____

CHAPTER 18

Nutrition and Metabolism

M ost of us love to eat, but do the foods we enjoy provide us with the basic food types necessary for good nutrition? The body, a finely tuned machine, requires a balance of carbohydrates, fats, proteins, vitamins, and minerals to function properly. These nutrients must be digested, absorbed, and circulated to cells constantly to accommodate the numerous activities that occur throughout the body. The use the body makes of foods once these processes are completed is called *metabolism*.

The liver plays a major role in the metabolism of food. It helps maintain a normal blood glucose level, removes toxins from the blood, processes blood immediately after it leaves the gastrointestinal tract, and initiates the first steps of protein and fat metabolism.

This chapter also discusses basal metabolic rate (BMR). The BMR is the rate at which food is catabolized under basal conditions. This test and the protein-bound iodine (PBI) are indirect measures of thyroid gland functioning. The total metabolic rate (TMR) is the amount of energy, expressed in calories, used by the body each day.

Finally, maintaining a constant body temperature is a function of the hypothalamus and a challenge for the metabolic mechanisms of the body. Review of this chapter is necessary to provide you with an understanding of the "fuel" (nutrition) requirements necessary to maintain this complex homeostatic machine—the body.

TOPICS FOR REVIEW

Before progressing to Chapter 19, you should be able to define and contrast catabolism and anabolism. Your review should include the metabolic roles of carbohydrates, fats, proteins, vitamins, and minerals. Your study should conclude with an understanding of the basal metabolic rate, physiological mechanisms that regulate body temperature, and the common metabolic and eating disorders.

METABOLIC FUNCTIONS OF THE LIVER

Fill in the blanks.

The liver plays an important role in the mechanical digestion of lipids because it secretes
(1) _____. It also produces two of the plasma proteins that play an essential
role in blood clotting. These two proteins are (2) _____ and
(3) _____. Additionally, liver cells store several substances, notably vitamins A and D and (4) _____. Finally, the liver is assisted by a unique structural feature of the blood vessels that supply it. This arrangement, known as the
(5) _____ _____
_____ , allows toxins to be removed from the bloodstream before nutrients
are distributed throughout the body.

NUTRIENT METABOLISM

Match each term with its corresponding definition. (Answers may be used more than once.)

_____ 6.	Used if cells have inadequate amounts of glucose to catabolize	A. Carbohydrate
_____ 7.	Preferred energy food	B. Fat
_____ 8.	Amino acids	C. Protein
_____ 9.	Fat soluble	D. Vitamins
_____ 10.	Required for nerve conduction	E. Minerals
_____ 11.	Glycolysis	
_____ 12.	Inorganic elements found naturally in the earth	
_____ 13.	Pyruvic acid	

Circle the term in each word group that does not belong.

14. Glycolysis	Citric acid cycle	ATP	Bile
15. Adipose	Amino acids	Triglycerides	Lipid
16. A	D	M	K
17. Iron	Proteins	Amino acids	Essential
18. Hydrocortisone	Insulin	Growth hormone	Epinephrine
19. Sodium	Calcium	Zinc	Folic acid
20. Thiamine	Niacin	Ascorbic acid	Riboflavin

▷ *If you had difficulty with this section, review pages 525-532.*

METABOLIC RATES

Circle the correct answer.

21. The rate at which food is catabolized under
    basal conditions is the:
    A. TMR
    B. PBI
    C. BMR
    D. ATP

22. The total amount of energy used by the body
    per day is the:
    A. TMR
    B. PBI
    C. BMR
    D. ATP

23. A/an _____ is the amount of energy needed to raise the temperature of 1 gram of water 1° Celsius.
    A. Calorie
    B. Kilocalorie
    C. ATP
    D. BMR

24. Which of the following is a factor when determining the BMR?
    A. Sex
    B. Age
    C. Size
    D. All of the above

25. Which of the following is a factor when determining the TMR?
    A. Exercise
    B. Food intake
    C. Environmental temperature
    D. All of the above

▷ *If you had difficulty with this section, review page 532.*

METABOLIC AND EATING DISORDERS

Match each description with its related term. Write the corresponding letter in the answer blank.

_____	26.	Insulin deficiency is a symptom of this disorder	A. BMR
_____	27.	Behavioral disorder characterized by chronic refusal to eat	B. Diabetes mellitus
_____	28.	An advanced form of PCM	C. Anorexia nervosa
_____	29.	Results from a deficiency of calories in general and protein in particular	D. Bulimia
_____	30.	Hypothyroidism will affect this measurement	E. Obesity
_____	31.	Abdominal bloating	F. PCM
_____	32.	Symptom of chronic overeating behavior	G. Marasmus
_____	33.	Behavioral disorder characterized by insatiable craving for food alternating with periods of self-deprivation	H. Ascites

▷ *If you had difficulty with this section, review pages 532-534.*

BODY TEMPERATURES

Circle the correct answer.

34. Over _____ of the energy released from food molecules during catabolism is converted to heat rather than being transferred to ATP.
    A. 20%
    B. 40%
    C. 60%
    D. 80%

35. Maintaining thermoregulation is a function of the:
    A. Thalamus
    B. Hypothalamus
    C. Thyroid
    D. Parathyroids

36. Transfer of heat energy to the skin, then the external environment is known as:
    A. Radiation
    B. Conduction
    C. Convection
    D. Evaporation

37. A flow of heat waves away from the blood is known as:
    A. Radiation
    B. Conduction
    C. Convection
    D. Evaporation

38. A transfer of heat energy to air that is continually flowing away from the skin is known as:
    A. Radiation
    B. Conduction
    C. Convection
    D. Evaporation

39. Heat that is absorbed by the process of water vaporization is called:
    A. Radiation
    B. Conduction
    C. Convection
    D. Evaporation

 If you had difficulty with this section, review pages 534-535.

ABNORMAL BODY TEMPERATURE

If the statement is true, write "T" in the answer blank. If the statement is false, correct the statement by circling the incorrect term and writing the correct term in the answer blank.

_____ 40. Pyrogens cause the thermostatic control centers of the hypothalamus to produce a fever.

_____ 41. Malignant hyperthermia is the inability to maintain a normal body temperature in extremely cold environments.

_____ 42. Frostbite is local damage to tissues caused by extremely low temperatures.

_____ 43. Heat exhaustion is characterized by body temperatures of 41° Celsius or higher.

_____ 44. Dantrium is used to prevent or relieve the effects of frostbite.

▷ *If you had difficulty with this section, review pages 535-537.*

UNSCRAMBLE THE WORDS

45. **L R I E V**

   ▢▢〇〇〇▢

46. **T A O B A L I C M S**

   ▢〇〇▢〇▢▢▢▢

47. **O M N I A**

   〇▢▢〇〇

48. **Y P U R C V I**

   〇▢▢▢▢〇▢

Take the circled letters, unscramble them, and fill in the solution.

How the magician paid his bills.

49. ▢▢▢▢▢▢▢▢▢▢▢▢▢▢

APPLYING WHAT YOU KNOW

50. Dr. Carey was concerned about Deborah. Her daily food intake provided fewer calories than her TMR. If this trend continues, what will be the result? If it continues over a long time, what eating disorder might Deborah develop?

51. Kathryn had been experiencing fatigue, and a blood test revealed that she was slightly anemic. What mineral will her doctor most likely prescribe? What dietary sources might you suggest that she emphasize in her daily intake?

52. Joe was training daily for an upcoming marathon. Three days before the 25-mile event, he suddenly quit his daily routine of jogging and switched to a diet high in carbohydrates. Why did Joe suddenly switch his routine of training?

53. Word Find

Find and circle 18 terms presented in this chapter. Words may be spelled top to bottom, bottom to top, right to left, left to right, or diagonally.

```
C  C  C  B  W  E  F  F  L  J  V  G  G  S
A  T  N  L  W  E  U  O  Z  I  E  L  I  B
R  K  K  P  Z  F  R  I  T  P  O  Y  K  L
B  Q  M  I  N  E  R  A  L  S  J  C  C  P
O  S  S  N  C  X  M  I  D  B  D  O  W  P
H  S  I  Y  O  I  T  X  H  I  N  L  S  N
Y  E  L  N  N  I  K  W  W  D  S  Y  N  S
D  G  O  S  O  W  T  I  U  E  H  S  C  N
R  M  B  Y  T  I  W  C  Z  N  N  I  A  A
A  R  A  Q  W  A  T  B  E  I  G  S  J  M
T  E  T  F  N  I  F  A  E  V  E  W  T  Y
E  V  A  P  O  R  A  T  I  O  N  D  T  E
S  I  C  N  E  S  O  P  I  D  A  O  F  E
H  L  Y  K  I  R  E  B  V  P  A  H  C  J
I  W  E  E  P  A  D  F  T  E  A  R  G  G
```

ATP	Conduction	Liver
Adipose	Convection	Minerals
BMR	Evaporation	Proteins
Bile	Fats	Radiation
Carbohydrates	Glycerol	TMR
Catabolism	Glycolysis	Vitamins

DID YOU KNOW?

The amount of energy required for a person to raise a 200-pound man 15 feet in the air is about the amount of energy in one large calorie.

NUTRITION/METABOLISM

Fill in the crossword puzzle.

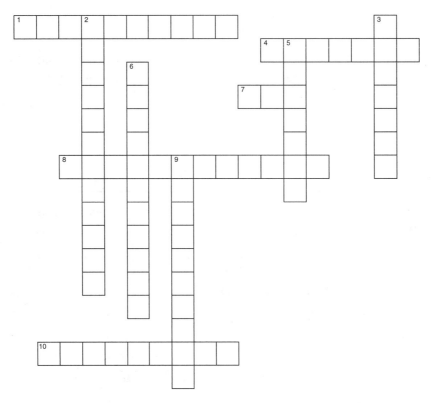

ACROSS

1.   Breaks food molecules down releasing stored energy
4.   Amount of energy needed to raise the temperature of one gram of water 1° Celsius
7.   Rate of metabolism when a person is lying down, but awake (abbreviation)
8.   A series of reactions that join glucose molecules together to form glycogen
10. Builds food molecules into complex substances

DOWN

2.   Occurs when food molecules enter cells and undergo many chemical changes there
3.   Organic molecule needed in small quantities for normal metabolism throughout the body
5.   Oxygen-using
6.   A unit of measure for heat, also known as a large calorie
9.   Takes place in the cytoplasm of a cell and changes glucose to pyruvic acid

CHECK YOUR KNOWLEDGE

Multiple Choice

Circle the correct answer.

1. The citric acid cycle changes acetyl CoA to:
   A. Oxygen
   B. Carbon dioxide
   C. Pyruvic acid
   D. Glucose

2. The anabolism of glucose produces which of the following?
   A. Glycogen
   B. Amino acid
   C. Rennin
   D. Starch

3. Which of the following is a major hormone in the body that aids carbohydrate metabolism?
   A. Oxytocin
   B. Epinephrine
   C. Insulin
   D. Growth hormone

4. The total metabolic rate is which of the following?
   A. The amount of fats a person consumes in a 24-hour period
   B. The same as the BMR
   C. The amount of energy expressed in calories used by the body per day
   D. Cannot be calculated

5. When your consumption of calories equals your TMR, your weight will do which of the following?
   A. Increase
   B. Remain the same
   C. Fluctuate
   D. Decrease

6. Which of the following is a normal glucose level?
   A. 40 to 80 mg/100 mL blood
   B. 80 to 120 mg/100 mL blood
   C. 100 to 140 mg/100 mL blood
   D. 180 to 220 mg/100 mL blood

7. When glucose is *not* available, the body will next catabolize which of the following energy sources?
   A. Fats
   B. Proteins
   C. Minerals
   D. Vitamins

8. Maintaining the homeostasis of the body temperature is the responsibility of which of the following?
   A. Hypothalamus
   B. Environmental condition in which we live
   C. Circulatory system
   D. None of the above

9. The liver plays an important role in the mechanical digestion of lipids because it secretes:
   A. Glucose molecules
   B. Bile
   C. Glycogen
   D. Citric acid

10. What is the primary molecule the body usually breaks down as an energy source?
    A. Amino acid
    B. Pepsin
    C. Maltose
    D. Glucose

Completion

Complete the following statements using the terms listed below. (Some words may be used more than once.)
Write the corresponding letter in the answer blank.

A. Vitamins
B. Insulin
C. Carbohydrates
D. Fats
E. Glycolysis
F. Metabolism

G. ATP
H. Sodium
I. Proteins
J. Citric acid cycle
K. Calcium
L. Glycogen loading

11. Proper nutrition requires the balance of the three basic food types: _____, _____, and _____.

12. The process that changes glucose to pyruvic acid is called _____.

13. Once glucose has been changed to pyruvic acid, another process in which pyruvic acid is changed to carbon dioxide takes place. This reaction is known as the _____.

14. A direct source of energy for doing cellular work is _____.

15. The only hormone that lowers blood glucose level is _____.

16. When cells have an inadequate amount of glucose to catabolize they will catabolize _____.

17. Some athletes consume large amounts of carbohydrates 2 to 3 days before an athletic event to store glycogen in skeletal muscles. This practice is called _____.

18. Organic molecules needed in small amounts for normal metabolism are _____.

19. Two minerals necessary for nerve conduction and contraction of muscle fibers are _____ and _____.

20. The "use of foods" is known as _____.

CHAPTER 19

The Urinary System

L iving produces wastes. Wherever people live, work, or play, wastes accumulate. To keep these areas healthy, there must be a method of disposing of these wastes such as the services provided by a sanitation department. Wastes also accumulate in your body. The conversion of food and gases into substances and energy necessary for survival results in waste products. A large percentage of these wastes is removed by the urinary system.

Two vital organs, the kidneys, cleanse the blood of the many waste products that are continually produced as a result of the metabolism of nutrients taken into the body cells. They eliminate these wastes in the form of urine.

Urine formation is the result of three processes: filtration, reabsorption, and secretion. These processes occur in successive portions of the microscopic units of the kidneys known as *nephrons*. The amount of urine produced by the nephrons is controlled primarily by the hormones ADH and aldosterone.

After urine is produced, it is drained from the renal pelvis by the ureters to flow into the bladder. The bladder then stores the urine until it is voided through the urethra.

If waste products are allowed to accumulate in the body, they soon become poisonous, a condition called *uremia*. A knowledge of the urinary system is necessary to understand how the body rids itself of waste and avoids toxicity.

TOPICS FOR REVIEW

Before progressing to Chapter 20, you should have an understanding of the structure and function of the organs of the urinary system. Your review should include knowledge of the nephron and its role in urine production. Your study should conclude with a review of the three main processes involved in urine production, the mechanisms that control urine volume, and the major renal and urinary disorders.

KIDNEYS

FORMATION OF URINE

Circle the correct answer.

1. The outermost portion of the kidney is known as the:
   A. Medulla
   B. Papilla
   C. Pelvis
   D. Pyramid
   E. Cortex

2. The saclike structure that surrounds the glomerulus is the:
   A. Renal pelvis
   B. Calyx
   C. Bowman capsule
   D. Cortex
   E. None of the above

3. The renal corpuscle is made up of the:
   A. Bowman capsule and proximal convoluted tubule
   B. Glomerulus and proximal convoluted tubule
   C. Bowman capsule and the distal convoluted tubule
   D. Glomerulus and the distal convoluted tubule
   E. Bowman capsule and the glomerulus

4. Which of the following functions is *not* performed by the kidneys?
   A. Help maintain homeostasis
   B. Remove wastes from the blood
   C. Produce ADH
   D. Remove electrolytes from the blood

5. _____ % of the glomerular filtrate is reabsorbed.
   A. 20
   B. 40
   C. 75
   D. 85
   E. 99

6. The glomerular filtration rate is _____ mL per minute.
   A. 1.25
   B. 12.5
   C. 125.0
   D. 1250.0
   E. None of the above

7. Glucose reabsorption begins in the:
   A. Henle loop
   B. Proximal convoluted tubule
   C. Distal convoluted tubule
   D. Glomerulus
   E. None of the above

8. Reabsorption does *not* occur in the:
   A. Henle loop
   B. Proximal convoluted tubule
   C. Distal convoluted tubule
   D. Collecting duct
   E. Calyx

9. The greater the amount of salt intake, the:
   A. Less salt is excreted in the urine
   B. More salt is reabsorbed
   C. More salt is excreted in the urine
   D. None of the above

10. Which one of the following substances is secreted by diffusion?
    A. Sodium ions
    B. Certain drugs
    C. Ammonia
    D. Hydrogen ions
    E. Potassium ions

11. Which of the following statements about ADH is *not* correct?
    A. It is stored by the pituitary gland.
    B. It makes the collecting ducts less permeable to water.
    C. It makes the distal convoluted tubules more permeable.
    D. It is produced by the hypothalamus.

12. Which of the following statements about aldosterone is *not* correct?
    A. It is secreted by the adrenal cortex.
    B. It is a water-retaining hormone.
    C. It is a salt-retaining hormone.
    D. All of the above are correct.

Match each descriptive phrase with its related structure. Write the corresponding letter in the answer blank.

_____ 13.	Functioning unit of the urinary system	A. Medulla
_____ 14.	Abnormal characteristic of urine	B. Cortex
_____ 15.	Normal characteristic of urine	C. Pyramids
_____ 16.	Outer part of the kidney	D. Papilla
_____ 17.	Together with the Bowman capsule forms the renal corpuscle	E. Pelvis
_____ 18.	Division of the renal pelvis	F. Calyx
_____ 19.	Cup-shaped top of a nephron	G. Nephrons
_____ 20.	Innermost end of a pyramid	H. Creatinine
_____ 21.	Extension of the proximal tubule	I. Albumin
_____ 22.	Triangular-shaped divisions of the medulla of the kidney	J. Bowman capsule
_____ 23.	An expansion of the upper end of a ureter	K. Glomerulus
_____ 24.	Inner portion of the kidney	L. Henle loop

▶ *If you had difficulty with this section, review pages 543-553.*

URETERS

URINARY BLADDER

URETHRA

Match each descriptive phrase with its related structure and write the corresponding letter in the answer blank.

A. Ureters   B. Bladder   C. Urethra

_____ 25. Lies between the urinary meatus and bladder

_____ 26. Rugae

_____ 27. Lowest part of the urinary tract

_____ 28. Lining membrane richly supplied with sensory nerve endings

_____ 29. Lies behind the pubic symphysis

_____ 30. Serves a dual function in the male

_____ 31. 1½ inches long in the female

_____ 32. Drain the renal pelvis

_____ 33. Surrounded by the prostate in the male

_____ 34. Consists of elastic fibers and involuntary muscle fibers

_____ 35. 10 to 12 inches long

_____ 36. Trigone

Fill in the blanks.

37. The physical, chemical, and microscopic examination of urine is termed
    _____.

38. The urinary tract is lined with _____ _____.

39. Urine specimens are often spun in a _____ to force suspended particles
    to the bottom of a test tube.

40. The absence of urine is known as _____.

41. Clinical studies have proven that improper catheterization techniques cause
    _____ in hospitalized patients.

42. In the male, the urethra serves a dual function: a passageway for urine and
    _____.

43. The external opening of the urethra is the _____
    _____.

▷ *If you had difficulty with this section, review pages 553-555.*

MICTURITION

Fill in the blanks.

The terms (44) _____, (45) _____, and
(46) _____ all refer to the passage of urine from the body or the emptying
of the bladder. The sphincters guard the bladder. The (47) _____
_____ _____ is the sphincter located at
the bladder (48) _____ and is involuntary. The external urethral sphincter
encircles the (49) _____ and is under
(50) _____ control. As the bladder fills, nervous impulses are transmitted to
the spinal cord and an (51) _____ is initiated. Urine then enters the
(52) _____ to be eliminated. Urinary
(53) _____ is a condition in which no urine is voided. Urinary
(54) _____ is when the kidneys do not produce any urine, but the bladder
retains its ability to empty itself. The term (55) _____
_____ is often used to describe the type of urine loss associated with laugh-
ing, coughing, or heavy lifting.

▷ *If you had difficulty with this section, review pages 554-556.*

RENAL AND URINARY DISORDERS

Match each descriptive phrase with its related disorder. Write the corresponding letter in the answer blank.

_____ 56. Urine backs up into the kidneys causing swelling of the renal pelvis and calyces

_____ 57. Kidney stones develop

_____ 58. Intermittent dribbling of urine

_____ 59. Blood in the urine

_____ 60. Inflammation of the bladder

_____ 61. Inflammation of the renal pelvis and connective tissues of the kidney

_____ 62. An abrupt reduction in kidney function characterized by oliguria and a sharp rise in nitrogenous compounds in the blood

_____ 63. Progressive condition resulting from gradual loss of nephrons

_____ 64. Intense kidney pain caused by obstruction of the ureters by large kidney stones

_____ 65. Most common form of kidney disease caused by a delayed immune response to streptococcal infection

_____ 66. Albumin in the urine

_____ 67. Inflammation of the urethra that commonly results from bacterial infection

A.   Pyelonephritis

B.   Renal colic

C.   Renal calculi

D.   Acute glomerulonephritis

E.   Proteinuria

F.   Hematuria

G.   Overflow incontinence

H.   Acute renal failure

I.   Hydronephrosis

J.   Chronic renal failure

K.   Cystitis

L.   Urethritis

▶ *If you had difficulty with this section, review pages 556-562.*

UNSCRAMBLE THE WORDS

68. **A Y X L C**

69. **G V N O I D I**

70. **A L P A L I P**

71. **S G U L L O U M R E**

Take the circled letters, unscramble them, and fill in the solution.

What Betty saw while cruising down the Nile.

72.

APPLYING WHAT YOU KNOW

73. John suffered from low levels of ADH. What primary urinary symptom would he notice?

74. Bud was in a diving accident and his spinal cord was severed. He was paralyzed from the waist down and as a result was incontinent. His physician, Dr. Welch, was concerned about the continuous residual urine buildup. What was the reason for concern?

75. Mrs. Lynch had a prolonged surgical procedure and experienced problems with urinary retention postoperatively. A urinary catheter was inserted into her bladder for the elimination of urine. Several days later Mrs. Lynch developed cystitis. What might be a possible cause of this diagnosis?

76. Mr. Dietz, an accident victim, was admitted to the hospital several hours ago. His chart indicates that he had been hemorrhaging at the scene of the accident. Nurse Petersen has been closely monitoring his urinary output and has noted that it has dropped to 10 mL/hr. (The normal urine output for a healthy adult is approximately 30 to 60 mL/hr.) What might explain this drop in urine output?

77. **Word Find**

Find and circle 18 terms presented in this chapter. Words may be spelled top to bottom, bottom to top, right to left, left to right, or diagonally.

```
H  N  O  I  T  I  R  U  T  C  I  M  N  M  Y
V  E  Q  N  G  A  L  L  I  P  A  P  S  E  S
T  P  M  C  O  L  D  U  J  Y  S  I  N  D  D
L  H  G  O  X  I  O  W  C  G  V  D  I  U  J
C  R  F  N  D  B  T  M  T  L  I  M  B  K  L
P  O  O  T  X  I  C  A  E  K  A  P  X  L  D
Q  N  U  I  E  G  A  P  R  R  T  C  W  A  O
B  J  R  N  T  T  L  Y  T  U  Y  G  D  M
S  D  E  E  R  G  Y  P  Y  V  L  L  P  H  Z
I  H  T  N  O  U  X  W  D  S  X  I  U  J  G
M  X  E  C  C  Y  S  T  I  T  I  S  F  S  Q
J  O  R  E  D  D  A  L  B  U  E  S  G  B  S
Y  I  S  E  B  V  L  L  B  H  V  Q  L  U  L
```

ADH	Filtration	Micturition
Bladder	Glomerulus	Nephron
Calculi	Hemodialysis	Papilla
Calyx	Incontinence	Pelvis
Cortex	Kidney	Pyramids
Cystitis	Medulla	Ureters

DID YOU KNOW?

If the tubules in a kidney were stretched out and untangled, they would measure 70 miles in length.

One out of every six men will develop prostate cancer in his lifetime, but only one man in every 35 will die from it.

URINARY SYSTEM

Fill in the crossword puzzle.

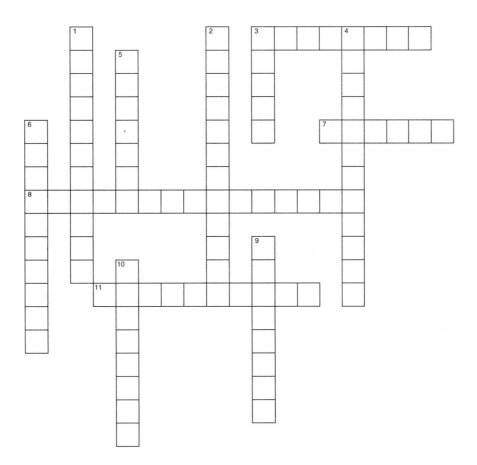

ACROSS

3. Bladder infection
7. Absence of urine
8. Passage of a tube into the bladder to withdraw urine
11. Network of blood capillaries tucked into Bowman's capsule

DOWN

1. Urination
2. Ultrasound generator used to break up kidney stones
3. Division of the renal pelvis
4. Voiding involuntarily
5. Area on posterior bladder wall free of rugae
6. Glucose in the urine
9. Large amount of urine
10. Scanty urine

CHECK YOUR KNOWLEDGE

Multiple Choice

Circle the correct answer.

1. Which of the following is true of urinary catheterization?
   A. It can be used to treat retention.
   B. It requires aseptic technique.
   C. It can lead to cystitis.
   D. All of the above are true.

2. Which of the following processes are used by the artificial kidney to remove waste materials from blood?
   A. Pinocytosis
   B. Dialysis
   C. Catheterization
   D. Active transport

3. Failure of the kidneys to remove wastes from the blood will result in which of the following?
   A. Retention
   B. Anuria
   C. Incontinence
   D. Uremia

4. Hydrogen ions are transferred from blood into the urine during which of the following processes?
   A. Secretion
   B. Filtration
   C. Reabsorption
   D. All of the above

5. Which of the following conditions would be expected in an infant under 2 years of age?
   A. Retention
   B. Cystitis
   C. Incontinence
   D. Anuria

6. Which of the following steps involved in urine formation allows the blood to retain most body nutrients?
   A. Secretion
   B. Filtration
   C. Reabsorption
   D. All of the above

7. Voluntary control of micturition is achieved by the action of which of the following?
   A. Internal urethral sphincter
   B. External urethral sphincter
   C. Trigone
   D. Bladder muscles

8. What is the structure that carries urine from the kidney to the bladder called?
   A. Urethra
   B. Bowman capsule
   C. Ureter
   D. Renal pelvis

9. What are the capillary loops contained within the Bowman capsule called?
   A. Convoluted tubules
   B. Glomeruli
   C. Henle loop limbs
   D. Collecting ducts

10. The triangular divisions of the medulla of the kidney are known as:
    A. Pyramids
    B. Papillae
    C. Calyces
    D. Nephrons

Matching

Match each term in column A with its corresponding description. (Only one answer is correct for each.)

Column A

_____ 11. Retention

_____ 12. Anuria

_____ 13. Cystitis

_____ 14. Micturition

_____ 15. Oliguria

_____ 16. Polyuria

_____ 17. Incontinence

_____ 18. Hematuria

_____ 19. Suppression

_____ 20. Reabsorption

Column B

A. Involuntary voiding

B. Movement of substance out of renal tubules into blood

C. Absence of urine

D. Urination

E. Bladder does not empty

F. Inflammation of the urinary bladder

G. Traces of blood in the urine

H. Large amount of urine

I. Kidneys not producing urine

J. Scanty amount of urine

URINARY SYSTEM

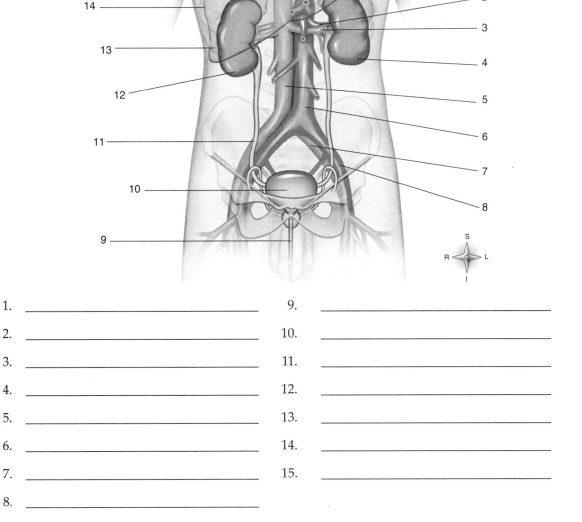

1. _____

2. _____

3. _____

4. _____

5. _____

6. _____

7. _____

8. _____

9. _____

10. _____

11. _____

12. _____

13. _____

14. _____

15. _____

KIDNEY

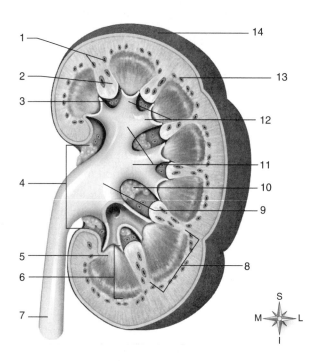

1. _____   8. _____

2. _____   9. _____

3. _____   10. _____

4. _____   11. _____

5. _____   12. _____

6. _____   13. _____

7. _____   14. _____

NEPHRON

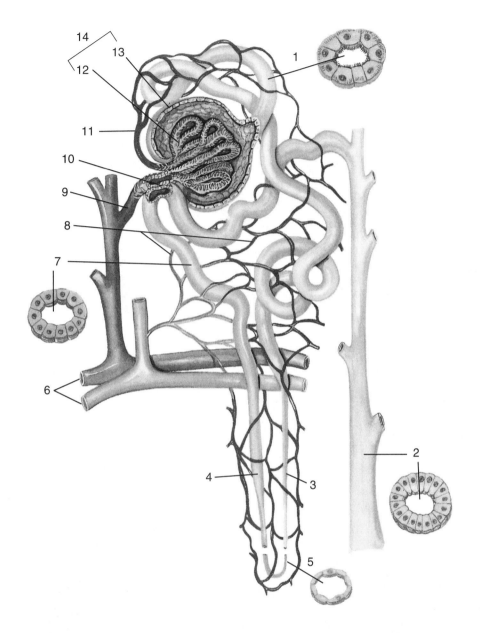

1. _____

2. _____

3. _____

4. _____

5. _____

6. _____

7. _____

8. _____

9. _____

10. _____

11. _____

12. _____

13. _____

14. _____

Fluid and Electrolyte Balance

Referring to the first chapter in your text, you will recall that survival depends on the body's ability to maintain or restore homeostasis. Specifically, *homeostasis* means that the body fluids remain constant within very narrow limits. These fluids are classified as either intracellular fluid (ICF) or extracellular fluid (ECF). As their names imply, intracellular fluid lies within the cells and extracellular fluid is located outside the cells. A balance between these two fluids is maintained by certain body mechanisms. They are (1) the adjustment of fluid output to fluid intake under normal circumstances; (2) the concentration of electrolytes in the extracellular fluid; (3) the capillary blood pressure; and finally, (4) the concentration of proteins in the blood.

Comprehension of how these mechanisms maintain and restore fluid balance is necessary for an understanding of the complexities of homeostasis and its relationship to the survival of the individual.

TOPICS FOR REVIEW

Before progressing to Chapter 21, you should review the types of body fluids and their subdivisions. Your study should include the mechanisms that maintain fluid balance and the nature and importance of electrolytes in body fluids. You should be able to give examples of common fluid imbalances, and have an understanding of the role of fluid and electrolyte balance in the maintenance of homeostasis.

BODY FLUIDS

Circle the correct answer.

1. The largest volume of water in the body by far lies (*inside* or *outside*) cells.

2. Interstitial fluid is (*intracellular* or *extracellular*).

3. Plasma is (*intracellular* or *extracellular*).

4. Obese people have a (*lower* or *higher*) water content per pound of body weight than thin people.

5. Infants have (*more* or *less*) water in comparison to body weight than adults of either sex.

6. There is a rapid (*increase* or *decline*) in the proportion of body water to body weight during the first 10 years of life.

7. The female body contains slightly (*more* or *less*) water per pound of weight.

8. In general, as age increases, the amount of water per pound of body weight (*increases* or *decreases*).

9. Excluding adipose tissue, approximately (*55%* or *85%*) of body weight is water.

10. The term (*fluid balance* or *fluid compartments*) means the volumes of ICF, IF, plasma, and the total volume of water in the body all remain relatively constant.

 If you had difficulty with this section, review pages 569-571.

MECHANISMS THAT MAINTAIN FLUID BALANCE

Circle the correct answer.

11. Which one of the following is *not* a positively charged ion?
    A. Chloride
    B. Calcium
    C. Sodium
    D. Potassium

12. Which one of the following is *not* a negatively charged ion?
    A. Chloride
    B. Bicarbonate
    C. Phosphate
    D. Sodium

13. The most abundant electrolyte in blood plasma is:
    A. NaCl
    B. KMg
    C. HCO_3
    D. HPO_4
    E. $CaPO_4$

14. What source contributes the least amount of water in the body?
    A. Water in foods that are eaten
    B. Ingested liquids
    C. Water formed from catabolism
    D. None of the above

15. The greatest amount of water lost from the body comes from the:
    A. Lungs
    B. Skin by diffusion
    C. Skin by sweat
    D. Feces
    E. Kidneys

16. Which one of the following is *not* a major factor that influences extracellular and intracellular fluid volumes?
    A. Concentration of electrolytes in the extracellular fluid
    B. Capillary blood pressure
    C. Concentration of proteins in blood
    D. All of the above are important factors

17. The fluid output source that changes the most is:
    A. Water loss in the feces
    B. Water loss from the skin
    C. Water loss via the lungs
    D. Water loss in the urine
    E. None of the above

18. The chief regulators of sodium within the body are the:
    A. Lungs
    B. Sweat glands
    C. Kidneys
    D. Large intestine
    E. None of the above

19. Which of the following is *not* correct?
    A. Fluid output must equal fluid intake.
    B. ADH controls salt reabsorption in the kidney.
    C. Water follows sodium.
    D. Renal tubule regulation of salt and water is the most important factor in determining urine volume.
    E. All of the above are correct.

20. Diuretics work on all but which one of the following?
    A. Proximal tubule
    B. Henle loop
    C. Distal tubule
    D. Collecting ducts
    E. Diuretics work on all of the above

21. Of all the sodium-containing secretions, the one with the largest volume is:
    A. Saliva
    B. Gastric secretions
    C. Bile
    D. Pancreatic juice
    E. Intestinal secretions

22. The higher the capillary blood pressure, the
_____the amount of interstitial fluid.
    A. Smaller
    B. Larger
    C. There is no relationship between capillary
       blood pressure and volume of interstitial
       fluid.

23. An increase in capillary blood pressure will
lead to _____ in blood volume.
    A. An increase
    B. A decrease
    C. No change
    D. None of the above

24. Which one of the fluid compartments varies the
most in volume?
    A. Intracellular
    B. Interstitial
    C. Extracellular
    D. Plasma

If the statement is true, write "T" in the answer blank. If the statement is false, correct the statement by circling the incorrect term and writing the correct term in the answer blank.

_____ 25. The three sources of fluid intake are the liquids we drink, the foods we eat, and water formed by the anabolism of foods.

_____ 26. The body maintains fluid balance mainly by changing the volume of urine excreted to match changes in the volume of fluid intake.

_____ 27. Some output of fluid will occur as long as life continues.

_____ 28. Glucose is an example of an electrolyte.

_____ 29. Where sodium goes, water soon follows.

_____ 30. Excess aldosterone leads to hypovolemia.

_____ 31. Diuretics have their effect on glomerular function.

_____ 32. Typical daily intake and output totals should be approximately 1200 mL.

_____ 33. Bile is a sodium-containing internal secretion.

_____ 34. The average daily diet contains about 500 mEq of sodium.

▶ *If you had difficulty with this section, review pages 571-578.*

FLUID IMBALANCES

Fill in the blanks.

(35) _____ is the fluid imbalance seen most often. In this condition, interstitial fluid volume (36) _____ first, but eventually, if treatment has not been given, intracellular fluid and plasma volumes (37) _____.

(38) _____ can also occur, but is much less common. Giving

(39) _____ _____ too rapidly or in too large amounts can put too heavy a burden on the (40) _____.

(41) _____ describes a blood sodium level above 145 mEq/L.

(42) _____ is a clinical term used to describe blood potassium levels above 5.1 mEq/L.

▶ *If you had difficulty with this section, review pages 577-580.*

UNSCRAMBLE THE WORDS

43. **M D E E A**

□○□□○□

44. **D F I L U**

□○□□□

45. **N I O**

□○□

46. **S O U I T N V A R E N**

□□□□□○□□□○□

Take the circled letters, unscramble them, and fill in the solution.

What Gary's dad disliked most about his music.

47. □□□□□□

APPLYING WHAT YOU KNOW

48. Mrs. Titus was asked to keep an accurate record of her fluid intake and output. She was concerned because the two did not balance. What is a possible explanation for this?

49. Nurse Briker was caring for a patient who was receiving diuretics. What special nursing implications should be followed for patients being given this therapy?

50. Jack Sprat was 6'5" and weighed 185 lbs. His wife was 5'6" and weighed 185 lbs. Whose body contained more water?

51. Word Find

Find and circle 12 terms presented in this chapter. Words may be spelled top to bottom, bottom to top, right to left, left to right, or diagonally.

```
S  T  V  H  O  M  E  O  S  T  A  S  I  S  H
I  E  D  E  M  A  S  Q  A  L  P  U  E  G  L
M  M  L  U  F  L  U  I  D  O  Y  O  I  S  L
W  S  B  E  A  E  C  O  L  D  P  N  I  E  R
L  I  T  A  C  V  S  H  Q  O  C  E  H  B  C
L  L  X  J  L  T  E  A  W  Y  B  V  Q  Q  O
I  O  O  P  E  A  R  U  C  T  C  A  A  R  I
N  B  H  R  X  S  N  O  I  I  P  R  T  C  N
S  A  O  X  M  G  J  C  L  N  J  T  B  A  H
I  N  X  X  D  V  U  D  E  Y  K  N  Y  O  C
E  A  A  J  Q  D  I  U  R  E  T  I  C  S  X
I  F  C  J  A  M  P  V  E  N  B  E  Y  F  W
V  F  K  T  Q  X  R  M  D  D  S  I  V  O  T
E  T  T  Z  N  T  R  P  X  I  M  L  J  F  I
S  W  Y  A  P  V  Q  N  S  K  T  K  W  B  P
```

Aldosterone	Edema	Imbalance
Anabolism	Electrolyte	Intravenous
Catabolism	Fluid	Ions
Diuretics	Homeostasis	Kidney

DID YOU KNOW?

The best fluid replacement drink is 1/4 tsp. of table salt added to 1 quart of water.

If all of the water were drained from the body of an average 160-pound man, the body would weigh 64 pounds.

FLUID/ELECTROLYTES

Fill in the crossword puzzle.

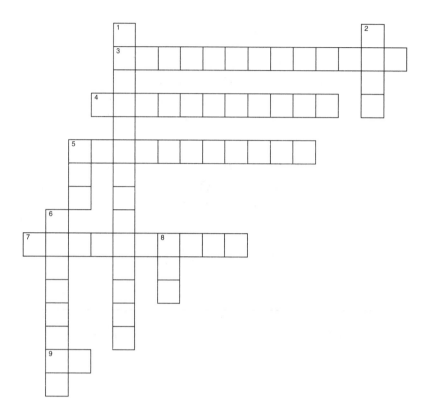

ACROSS

3. Result of rapidly given intravenous fluids
4. Result of large loss of body fluids
5. Compound that dissociates in solution into ions
7. To break up
9. A subdivision of extracellular fluid (abbreviation)

DOWN

1. Organic substance that doesn't dissociate in solution
2. Dissociated particles of an electrolyte that carry an electrical charge
5. Fluid outside cells (abbreviation)
6. "Causing urine"
8. Fluid inside cells (abbreviation)

CHECK YOUR KNOWLEDGE

Multiple Choice

Circle the correct answer.

1. Which of the following statements, if any, is *false*?
    A. The more fat present in the body, the more total water content per unit of weight.
    B. The body weight of infants is composed of a higher percentage of water in comparison with the body weight of adults.
    C. As age increases, the amount of water per pound of body weight decreases.
    D. All of the above statements are true.

2. Avenues of fluid output include which of the following?
    A. Skin
    B. Lungs
    C. Kidneys
    D. All of the above

3. Excessive water loss and fluid imbalance can result from which of the following?
    A. Diarrhea
    B. Vomiting
    C. Severe burns
    D. All of the above

4. What factor is primarily responsible for moving water from interstitial fluid into blood?
    A. Aldosterone secretions
    B. Pressure in blood capillaries
    C. Protein concentration of blood plasma
    D. Antidiuretic hormone secretions

5. What is the chief regulator of sodium levels in body fluids?
    A. Kidney
    B. Intestine
    C. Blood
    D. Lung

6. If blood sodium concentration decreases, what is the effect on blood volume?
    A. Increases
    B. Decreases
    C. Remains the same
    D. None of the above

7. Which of the following is true of body water?
    A. It is obtained from the liquids we drink.
    B. It is obtained from the foods we eat.
    C. It is formed by the catabolism of food.
    D. All of the above are true.

8. Edema may result from which of the following?
    A. Retention of electrolytes
    B. Decreased blood pressure
    C. Increased concentration of blood plasma proteins
    D. All of the above

9. The most abundant and most important positive plasma ion is which of the following?
    A. Sodium
    B. Chloride
    C. Calcium
    D. Oxygen

10. Which of the following is true when extracellular fluid volume decreases?
    A. Aldosterone secretion increases.
    B. Kidney tubule reabsorption of sodium increases.
    C. Urine volume decreases.
    D. All of the above are true.

Completion

Choose from the words below to complete the following statements. Write the corresponding letter in the answer blank.

A. Aldosterone
B. Edema
C. Proteins
D. Decreases
E. Diuretic

F. Electrolytes
G. Positive
H. Antidiuretic hormone
I. Dehydration
J. Extracellular fluid

K. Plasma
L. Urine
M. Interstitial fluid
N. Fluid balance

11. Any drug that promotes or stimulates the production of urine is called a _____.

12. The presence of abnormally large amounts of fluid in the intercellular tissue spaces of the body is called _____.

13. Water located outside of cells is called _____. It can be divided into two categories. If located in the spaces between the cells, it is called _____; and if located in blood vessels, it is called _____.

14. Compounds such as sodium chloride that form ions when placed in solution are called _____.

15. When the adrenal cortex increases its secretion of aldosterone, urine volume _____.

16. Most fluids leave the body in the form of _____.

17. When fluid output is greater than fluid intake, _____ occurs.

18. How much water moves into blood from interstitial fluid depends largely on the concentration of _____ present in blood plasma. These substances act as a water-pulling or water-holding force.

19. Urine volume is regulated primarily by a hormone secreted by the posterior lobe of the pituitary gland called _____ and by a hormone secreted by the adrenal gland called _____.

20. Homeostasis of fluids is also known as _____.

CHAPTER 21

Acid-Base Balance

I t has been established in previous chapters that equilibrium between intracellular and extracellular fluid volume must exist for homeostasis to be maintained. Equally important to homeostasis is the chemical acid-base balance of the body fluids. The degree of acidity or alkalinity of a body fluid is expressed in pH value. The neutral point, where a fluid would be neither acid nor alkaline, is pH 7. Increasing acidity is expressed as less than 7, and increasing alkalinity as greater than 7. Examples of body fluids that are acidic are gastric juice (1.6) and urine (6.0). Blood, on the other hand, is considered alkaline with a pH of 7.45.

Buffers are substances that prevent a sharp change in the pH of a fluid when an acid or base is added to it. Buffers are just one of several mechanisms that constantly monitor the pH of fluids in the body. If, for any reason, these mechanisms do not function properly, a pH imbalance occurs. The two general types of imbalances are known as *alkalosis* and *acidosis*.

Maintaining the acid-base balance of body fluids is a matter of vital importance. If this balance varies even slightly, necessary chemical and cellular reactions cannot occur. Your review of this chapter is necessary to understand the delicate acid-base balance that is necessary for survival.

TOPICS FOR REVIEW

Before progressing to Chapter 22, you should have an understanding of the pH of body fluids and the mechanisms that control the pH of these fluids in the body. Your study should conclude with a review of the metabolic and respiratory types of pH imbalances.

pH OF THE BODY

Identify each of the circumstances or substances as acid or base. Write the corresponding letter in the answer blank.

A. Acid   B. Base

_____ 1.   Lower concentration of hydrogen ions than hydroxide ions
_____ 2.   Higher concentration of hydrogen ions than hydroxide ions
_____ 3.   Gastric juice
_____ 4.   Saliva
_____ 5.   Arterial blood
_____ 6.   Venous blood
_____ 7.   Baking soda
_____ 8.   Beer
_____ 9.   Ammonia
_____ 10.   Sea water

▶ *If you had difficulty with this section, review pages 587-588.*

MECHANISMS THAT CONTROL THE pH OF BODY FLUIDS

Circle the correct answer.

11. When carbon dioxide enters the blood, it reacts with the enzyme carbonic anhydrase to form:
    A. Sodium bicarbonate
    B. Water and carbon dioxide
    C. Ammonium chloride
    D. Bicarbonate ion
    E. Carbonic acid

12. The lungs remove _____ liters of carbonic acid each day.
    A. 10.0
    B. 15.0
    C. 20.0
    D. 25.0
    E. 30.0

13. When a buffer reacts with a strong acid, it changes the strong acid to a:
    A. Weak acid
    B. Strong base
    C. Weak base
    D. Water
    E. None of the above

14. Which one of the following is *not* a change in the blood that results from the buffering of fixed acids in tissue capillaries?
    A. The amount of carbonic acid increases slightly.
    B. The amount of bicarbonate in blood decreases.
    C. The hydrogen ion concentration of blood increases slightly.
    D. The blood pH decreases slightly.
    E. All of the above are changes that result from the buffering of fixed acids in tissue capillaries.

15. The most abundant acid in body fluids is:
    A. HCl
    B. Lactic acid
    C. Carbonic acid
    D. Acetic acid
    E. Sulfuric acid

16. The normal ratio of sodium bicarbonate to carbonic acid in arterial blood is:
    A. 5:1
    B. 10:1
    C. 15:1
    D. 20:1
    E. None of the above

17. Which of the following would *not* be a consequence of holding your breath?
    A. The amount of carbonic acid in the blood would increase.
    B. The blood pH would decrease.
    C. The body would develop an alkalosis.
    D. No carbon dioxide could leave the body.

18. The most effective regulators of blood pH are:
    A. The lungs
    B. The kidneys
    C. Buffers
    D. None of the above

19. The pH of the urine may be as low as:
    A. 1.6
    B. 2.5
    C. 3.2
    D. 4.8
    E. 7.4

20. In the distal tubule cells, the product of the reaction aided by carbonic anhydrase is:
    A. Water
    B. Carbon dioxide
    C. Water and carbon dioxide
    D. Hydrogen ions
    E. Carbonic acid

21. In the distal tubule, _____ leaves the tubule cells and enters the blood capillaries.
    A. Carbon dioxide
    B. Water
    C. HCO_3
    D. NaH_2PO_4
    E. $NaHCO_3$

If the statement is true, write "T" in the answer blank. If the statement is false, correct the statement by circling the incorrect term and writing the correct term in the answer blank.

_____ 22. The body has three mechanisms for regulating the pH of its fluids. They are the heart mechanism, the respiratory mechanism, and the urinary mechanism.

_____ 23. Buffers consist of two kinds of substances and therefore are often called *duobuffers*.

_____ 24. Black coffee and cola are acidic on the pH scale.

_____ 25. Some athletes have adopted a technique called *bicarbonate loading*, ingesting large amounts of sodium bicarbonate ($NaHCO_3$) to counteract the effects of lactic acid buildup.

_____ 26. Anything that causes an excessive increase in respiration will, in time, produce acidosis.

_____ 27. Venous blood has a higher pH than arterial blood.

_____ 28. More acids than bases are usually excreted by the kidneys because more acids than bases usually enter the blood.

_____ 29. Blood levels of sodium bicarbonate can be regulated by the lungs.

_____ 30. Blood levels of carbonic acid can be regulated by the kidneys.

▶ *If you had difficulty with this section, review pages 588-594.*

METABOLIC AND RESPIRATORY DISTURBANCES

Match each numbered circumstance with its resulting condition. Write the corresponding letter in the answer blank.

_____ 31. Vomiting

_____ 32. Result of untreated diabetes

_____ 33. Chloride-containing solution

_____ 34. Bicarbonate deficit

_____ 35. Occurs during emesis and may result in metabolic alkalosis

_____ 36. Bicarbonate excess

_____ 37. Rapid breathing

_____ 38. Carbonic acid excess

_____ 39. Carbonic acid deficit

_____ 40. Glucophage

A. Metabolic acidosis

B. Metabolic alkalosis

C. Respiratory acidosis

D. Respiratory alkalosis

E. Emesis

F. Normal saline

G. Uncompensated metabolic acidosis

H. Hyperventilation

I. HCl loss

J. Antidiabetic medication

▶ *If you had difficulty with this section, review pages 594-597.*

APPLYING WHAT YOU KNOW

41. Holly was pregnant and experienced repeated vomiting episodes throughout the day for several days in a row. Her doctor became concerned, admitted her to the hospital, and began intravenous administrations of normal saline. How will this help Holly?

42. Cara had a minor bladder infection. She had heard that this is often the result of the urine being less acidic than necessary and that she should drink cranberry juice to correct the acid problem. She had no cranberry juice, so she decided to substitute orange juice. Why would this substitution not be effective in correcting the acid problem?

43. Mr. Shearer has frequent bouts of hyperacidity of the stomach. Which will assist in neutralizing the acid more promptly: milk or milk of magnesia?

44.   Word Find

Find and circle 18 terms presented in this chapter. Words may be spelled top to bottom, bottom to top, right to left, left to right, or diagonally.

```
S  I  S  A  T  S  O  E  M  O  H  P  R  G
E  C  N  A  L  A  B  D  I  U  L  F  E  F
T  S  Y  E  N  D  I  K  W  T  I  K  A  J
Y  D  M  N  D  E  J  W  L  P  T  D  J  I
L  D  N  O  L  H  V  W  O  U  H  D  O  I
O  V  E  R  H  Y  D  R  A  T  I  O  N  S
R  E  I  E  E  D  E  M  A  U  R  O  R  Q
T  L  M  T  C  R  U  L  R  F  S  E  O  Y
C  C  U  S  Z  A  W  E  K  A  T  N  I  X
E  O  Z  O  T  T  A  N  A  U  N  M  F
L  F  K  D  P  I  O  I  W  W  Q  L  G  Q
E  N  I  L  C  O  O  H  O  W  S  B  X  S
N  J  X  A  L  N  F  S  U  N  L  J  J  J
O  C  U  V  S  A  L  G  T  I  S  C  Z  X
N  I  Z  L  L  D  Y  X  Q  Q  K  D  C  D
```

ADH	Edema	Nonelectrolytes
Aldosterone	Electrolytes	Output
Anions	Fluid balance	Overhydration
Cations	Homeostasis	Sodium
Dehydration	Intake	Thirst
Diuretic	Kidneys	Water

DID YOU KNOW?

During the 19th century, English ships that were at sea for many months at a time carried limes onboard to feed the sailors to protect them from developing scurvy. American ships carried cranberries for this purpose.

ACID/BASE BALANCE

Fill in the crossword puzzle.

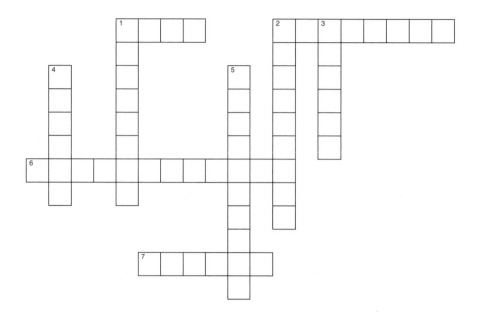

ACROSS

1. Substance with a pH lower than 7.0
2. Acid-base imbalance
6. Results from the excessive metabolism of fats in uncontrolled diabetics (two words)
7. Vomitus

DOWN

1. Substance with a pH higher than 7.0
2. Serious complication of vomiting
3. Emetic
4. Prevents a sharp change in the pH of fluids
5. Released as a waste product from working muscles (two words)

CHECK YOUR KNOWLEDGE

Multiple Choice

Circle the correct answer.

1. What happens as blood flows through lung capillaries?
   A. Carbonic acid in blood decreases.
   B. Hydrogen ions in blood decrease.
   C. Blood pH increases from venous to arterial blood.
   D. All of the above are true.

2. Which of the following organs is considered the most effective regulator of blood carbonic acid levels?
   A. Kidneys
   B. Intestines
   C. Lungs
   D. Stomach

3. Which of the following organs is considered the most effective regulator of blood pH?
   A. Kidneys
   B. Intestines
   C. Lungs
   D. Stomach

4. What is the pH of the blood?
   A. 7.00 to 8.00
   B. 6 25 to 7.45
   C. 7.65 to 7.85
   D. 7.35 to 7.45

5. If the ratio of sodium bicarbonate to carbonate ions is lowered (perhaps 10 to 1) and blood pH is also lowered, what is the condition called?
   A. Uncompensated metabolic acidosis
   B. Uncompensated metabolic alkalosis
   C. Compensated metabolic acidosis
   D. Compensated metabolic alkalosis

6. If a person hyperventilates for an extended time, which of the following will probably develop?
   A. Metabolic acidosis
   B. Metabolic alkalosis
   C. Respiratory acidosis
   D. Respiratory alkalosis

7. What happens when lactic acid dissociates in the blood?
   A. H+ is added to blood.
   B. pH is lowered.
   C. Acidosis results.
   D. All of the above happen.

8. Which of the following is true of metabolic alkalosis?
   A. It occurs in the case of prolonged vomiting.
   B. It results when the bicarbonate ion is present in excess.
   C. Therapy includes intravenous administration of normal saline.
   D. All of the above are true.

9. Which of the following is a characteristic of a buffer system in the body?
   A. It prevents drastic changes from occurring in body pH.
   B. It picks up both hydrogen and hydroxide ions.
   C. It is exemplified by the bicarbonate-carbonic acid system.
   D. All of the above are true.

10. In the presence of a strong acid (HCl), which of the following is true?
    A. Sodium bicarbonate will react to produce carbonic acid + sodium chloride.
    B. Sodium bicarbonate will react to produce more sodium bicarbonate.
    C. Carbonic acid will react to produce sodium bicarbonate.
    D. Carbonic acid will react to form more carbonic acid.

Matching

Match each description in column A with its corresponding term in column B. (Only one answer is correct for each.)

Column A

_____ 11. pH lower than 7.0

_____ 12. pH higher than 7.0

_____ 13. Prevent sharp pH changes

_____ 14. Decrease in respirations

_____ 15. Increase in respirations

_____ 16. Bicarbonate deficit

_____ 17. Bicarbonate excess

_____ 18. "Fixed" acid

_____ 19. Enzyme found in red blood cells

_____ 20. Lower-than-normal ratio of sodium bicarbonate to carbonic acid

Column B

A.   Metabolic acidosis

B.   Metabolic alkalosis

C.   Alkaline solution

D.   Lactic acid

E.   Respiratory acidosis

F.   Respiratory alkalosis

G.   Acidic solution

H.   Uncompensated metabolic acidosis

I.   Buffers

J.   Carbonic anhydrase

CHAPTER 22

The Reproductive Systems

The reproductive system consists of those organs that participate in perpetuating the species. It is a unique body system in that its organs differ between the two sexes, and yet the goal of creating a new being is the same for each gender. Of interest also is the fact that this system is the only one not necessary to the survival of the individual, and yet survival of the species depends on the proper functioning of the reproductive organs.

The male reproductive system is divided into the external genitals, the testes, the duct system, and accessory glands. The testes, or gonads, are considered essential organs because they produce the sex cells, sperm, which join with the female sex cells, ova, to form a new human being. They also secrete the male sex hormone, testosterone, which is responsible for the physical transformation of a boy to a man. Sperm are formed in the testes by the seminiferous tubules. From there they enter a long narrow duct, the epididymis. They continue onward through the vas deferens into the ejaculatory duct, down the urethra, and out of the body. Throughout this journey, various glands secrete substances that add motility to the sperm and create a chemical environment conducive to reproduction.

The female reproductive system is truly extraordinary and diverse. It produces ova, receives the penis and sperm during intercourse, is the site of conception, houses and nourishes the embryo during prenatal development, and nourishes the infant after birth. Because of its diversity, the physiology of the female is generally considered to be more complex than that of the male. Much of the activity of this system revolves around the menstrual cycle and the monthly preparation that the female undergoes for a possible pregnancy.

The organs of the reproductive systems are divided into essential organs and accessory organs of reproduction. The essential organs of the female are the ovaries. Just as with the male, the essential organs of the female are referred to as the *gonads*. The gonads of both sexes produce the sex cells. In the male, the gonads produce the sperm and in the female they produce the ova. The gonads are also responsible for producing the hormones in each gender that are necessary for development of the secondary sex characteristics.

The menstrual cycle of the female typically covers a period of 28 days. Each cycle consists of three phases: the menstrual period, the proliferative phase, and the secretory phase. Changes in the blood levels of the hormones that are responsible for the menstrual cycle also cause physical and emotional changes in the female. Knowledge of these phenomena and this system, in both the male and the female, are necessary to complete your understanding of the reproductive system.

TOPICS FOR REVIEW

Before progressing to Chapter 23, you should familiarize yourself with the structure and function of the organs of the male and female reproductive systems. Your review should include emphasis on the gross and microscopic structure of the testes and the production of sperm and testosterone. Your study should continue by tracing the pathway of a sperm cell from formation to expulsion from the body.

You should then familiarize yourself with the structure and function of the organs of the female reproductive system. Your review should include emphasis on the development of mature ova from ovarian follicles, and should additionally concentrate on the phases and occurrences in a typical 28-day menstrual cycle. Finally, a review of the common disorders occurring in both male and female reproductive systems is necessary to complete the study of this chapter.

MALE REPRODUCTIVE SYSTEM
STRUCTURAL PLAN

Match each term on the left with its related term on the right. Write the corresponding letter in the answer blank.

Group A

_____ 1.	Testes	A.	Fertilized ovum
_____ 2.	Spermatozoa	B.	Accessory organ
_____ 3.	Ovum	C.	Male sex cell
_____ 4.	Penis	D.	Gonads
_____ 5.	Zygote	E.	Gamete

Group B

_____ 6.	Testes	A.	Cowper gland
_____ 7.	Bulbourethral	B.	Scrotum
_____ 8.	Asexual	C.	Essential organ
_____ 9.	External genital	D.	Single parent
_____ 10.	Prostate	E.	Accessory organ

▶ *If you had difficulty with this section, review pages 603-605.*

TESTES

Circle the correct answer.

11. The testes are surrounded by a tough membrane called the:
    A. Ductus deferens
    B. Tunica albuginea
    C. Septum
    D. Seminiferous membrane

12. The _____ lie near the septa that separate the lobules.
    A. Ductus deferens
    B. Sperm
    C. Interstitial cells
    D. Nerves

13. Sperm are found in the walls of the _____.
    A. Seminiferous tubule
    B. Interstitial cells
    C. Septum
    D. Blood vessels

14. The scrotum provides an environment that is approximately _____ for the testes.
    A. The same as the body temperature
    B. 5 degrees warmer than the body temperature
    C. 3 degrees warmer than the body temperature
    D. 3 degrees cooler than the body temperature

15. The _____ produce(s) testosterone.
    A. Seminiferous tubules
    B. Prostate gland
    C. Bulbourethral gland
    D. Pituitary gland
    E. Interstitial cells

16. The part of the sperm that contains genetic information that will be inherited is the:
    A. Tail
    B. Neck
    C. Middle piece
    D. Head
    E. Acrosome

17. Which one of the following is *not* a function of testosterone?
    A. It causes a deepening of the voice.
    B. It promotes the development of the male accessory organs.
    C. It has a stimulatory effect on protein catabolism.
    D. It causes greater muscular development and strength.

18. Sperm production is called:
    A. Spermatogonia
    B. Spermatids
    C. Spermatogenesis
    D. Spermatocyte

19. The section of the sperm that contains enzymes that enable it to break down the covering of the ovum and permit entry should contact occur is the:
    A. Acrosome
    B. Midpiece
    C. Tail
    D. Stem

Fill in the blanks.

The (20) _____ are the gonads of the male. From puberty on, the seminiferous tubules are continuously forming (21) _____. Any of these cells may join with the female sex cell, the (22) _____, to become a new human being. Another function of the testes is to secrete the male hormone (23) _____, which transforms a boy to a man. This hormone is secreted by the (24) _____ _____ of the testes. A good way to remember testosterone's functions is to think of it as "the (25) _____ hormone" and "the (26) _____ hormone."

▶ *If you had difficulty with this section, review pages 605-609.*

REPRODUCTIVE DUCTS
ACCESSORY OR SUPPORTIVE SEX GLANDS
EXTERNAL GENITALS

Match each description on the left with its corresponding term on the right. Write the letter in the answer blank.

_____ 27.	Continuation of ducts that start in the epididymis	A.	Epididymis
_____ 28.	Erectile tissue	B.	Ductus (vas) deferens
_____ 29.	Also known as *bulbourethral*	C.	Ejaculatory duct
_____ 30.	Narrow tube that lies along the top and behind the testes	D.	Prepuce
_____ 31.	Doughnut-shaped gland beneath the bladder	E.	Seminal vesicles
_____ 32.	Point where ductus (vas) deferens joins the duct from the seminal vesicle	F.	Prostate gland
_____ 33.	Mixture of sperm and secretions of accessory sex glands	G.	Cowper gland
_____ 34.	Contributes 60% of the seminal fluid volume	H.	Corpus spongiosum
_____ 35.	Removed during circumcision	I.	Semen
_____ 36.	External genitalia	J.	Scrotum

▶ *If you had difficulty with this section, review pages 609-611.*

DISORDERS OF THE MALE REPRODUCTIVE SYSTEM

Fill in the blanks.

37. Decreased sperm production is called _____.

38. Testes normally descend into the scrotum about _____ _____ before birth.

39. If a baby is born with undescended testes, a condition called _____ results.

40. A common noncancerous condition of the prostate in older men is known as _____ _____ _____.

41. _____ is a condition in which the foreskin fits so tightly over the glans that it cannot retract.

42. Failure to achieve an erection of the penis is called _____.

43. An accumulation of fluid in the scrotum is known as a _____.

44. An _____ _____ results when the intestines push through the weak area of the abdominal wall, which separates the abdominopelvic cavity from the scrotum.

45. The PSA test is a screening test for cancer of the _____.

▶ *If you had difficulty with this section, review pages 611-614.*

FEMALE REPRODUCTIVE SYSTEM
STRUCTURAL PLAN

Match the term on the left with the corresponding term on the right. Write the letter in the answer blank.

_____ 46. Ovaries   A. Genitals
_____ 47. Vagina   B. Accessory sex gland
_____ 48. Bartholin   C. Accessory duct
_____ 49. Vulva   D. Gonads
_____ 50. Ova   E. Sex cell

Identify each of the numbered structures as external or internal. Write the corresponding letter in the answer blank.

A. External structure   B. Internal structure

_____ 51.   Mons pubis
_____ 52.   Vagina
_____ 53.   Labia majora
_____ 54.   Uterine tubes
_____ 55.   Vestibule
_____ 56.   Clitoris
_____ 57.   Labia minora
_____ 58.   Ovaries

▶ *If you had difficulty with this section, review pages 614-617.*

OVARIES

Fill in the blanks.

The ovaries are the (59) _____ of the female. They have two main functions. The first is the production of the female sex cell. This process is called (60) _____. The specialized type of cell division that occurs during sexual cell reproduction is known as (61) _____. The ovum is the body's largest cell and has (62) _____ the number of chromosomes found in other body cells. At the time of (63) _____, the sex cells from both parents fuse and (64) _____ chromosomes are united. The second major function of the ovaries is to secrete the sex hormones (65) _____ and (66) _____. Estrogen is the sex hormone that causes the development and maintenance of the female (67) _____ _____ _____. Progesterone acts with estrogen to help initiate the (68) _____ _____ in girls entering (69) _____.

▶ *If you had difficulty with this section, review pages 614-617.*

FEMALE REPRODUCTIVE DUCTS

Match each of the numbered descriptions with its corresponding structure. Write the letter in the answer blank.

A. Uterine tubes   B. Uterus   C. Vagina

_____ 70.   Location of most ectopic pregnancies

_____ 71.   Lining known as *endometrium*

_____ 72.   Birth canal

_____ 73.   Site of menstruation

_____ 74.   Fringelike projections called *fimbriae*

_____ 75.   Consists of a body, fundus, and cervix

_____ 76.   Site of fertilization

_____ 77.   Also known as *oviduct*

_____ 78.   Entranceway for sperm

▶ *If you had difficulty with this section, review pages 617-618.*

ACCESSORY OR SUPPORTIVE SEX GLANDS
EXTERNAL GENITALS

Match each term on the left with its corresponding description on the right. Write the letter in the answer blank.

Group A

_____ 79.   Bartholin glands   A.   Colored area around the nipple

_____ 80.   Breasts   B.   Grapelike clusters of milk-secreting cells

_____ 81.   Alveoli   C.   Drain alveoli

_____ 82.   Lactiferous ducts   D.   Also known as *greater vestibular*

_____ 83.   Areola   E.   Composed primarily of fat tissue

Group B

_____ 84.   Mons pubis   A.   "Large lips"

_____ 85.   Labia majora   B.   Area between the vaginal opening and the anus

_____ 86.   Clitoris   C.   Surgical procedure

_____ 87.   Perineum   D.   Composed of erectile tissue

_____ 88.   Episiotomy   E.   Pad of fat over the symphysis pubis

▶ *If you had difficulty with this section, review pages 618-620.*

MENSTRUAL CYCLE

If the statement is true, write "T" in the answer blank. If the statement is false, correct the statement by circling the incorrect term and writing the correct term in the answer blank.

_____ 89. *Climacteric* is the scientific name for the beginning of the menses.

_____ 90. As a general rule, several ovum mature each month during the 30 to 40 years that a woman has menstrual periods.

_____ 91. Ovulation occurs 28 days before the next menstrual period begins.

_____ 92. The first day of ovulation is considered the first day of the cycle.

_____ 93. A woman's fertile period lasts only a few days out of each month.

_____ 94. The control of the menstrual cycle lies in the posterior pituitary gland.

Match the two hormones below to their corresponding descriptions. Write the letter in the answer blank.

A. FSH   B. LH

_____ 95. Ovulating hormone

_____ 96. Secreted during first days of menstrual cycle

_____ 97. Secreted after estrogen level of blood increases

_____ 98. Causes final maturation of follicle and ovum

_____ 99. Suppressed by birth control pills

▶ *If you had difficulty with this section, review pages 620-622.*

DISORDERS OF THE FEMALE REPRODUCTIVE SYSTEM

Match each numbered description to its corresponding disease or condition. Write the letter in the answer blank.

_____ 100. Often occurs as a result of an STD or a "yeast infection"
_____ 101. Benign tumor of smooth muscle and fibrous connective tissue; also known as a *fibroid tumor*
_____ 102. Yeast infection characterized by leukorrhea
_____ 103. Inflammation of an ovary
_____ 104. Benign lumps in one or both breasts
_____ 105. Venereal diseases
_____ 106. Results from pathogenic organisms transmitted from another person; for example, an STD
_____ 107. Painful menstruation
_____ 108. Asymptomatic in most women and nearly all men
_____ 109. Results from a hormonal imbalance rather than from an infection or disease condition
_____ 110. Screening test for cervical cancer
_____ 111. Causes blisters on the skin of the genitals; the blisters may disappear temporarily, but recur, especially as a result of stress

A. Candidiasis
B. Dysmenorrhea
C. Exogenous infections
D. DUB
E. Myoma
F. Vaginitis
G. Sexually transmitted diseases (STDs)
H. Oophoritis
I. Fibrocystic disease
J. Pap smear
K. Genital herpes
L. Trichomoniasis

▶ *If you had difficulty with this section, review pages 622-629.*

APPLYING WHAT YOU KNOW

112. Sam is going into the hospital for the surgical removal of his testes. As a result of this surgery, will Sam be impotent?

113. When baby Christopher was born, the pediatrician, Dr. Self, discovered that his left testicle had not descended into the scrotum. If this situation is not corrected soon, might baby Christopher be sterile or impotent?

114. Charlene contracted gonorrhea. By the time she made an appointment to see her doctor, it had spread to her abdominal organs. How is this possible when gonorrhea is a disease of the reproductive system?

115. Dr. Sullivan advised Mrs. Harlan to have a bilateral oophorectomy. Is this a sterilization procedure? Will she experience menopause?

116. Vicki had a total hysterectomy. Will she experience menopause?

117. Word Find

Find and circle 18 terms presented in this chapter. Words may be spelled top to bottom, bottom to top, right to left, left to right, or diagonally.

```
M  K  O  V  I  D  U  C  T  S  E  D  H  G
S  E  I  R  A  V  O  I  F  U  T  G  L  L
I  N  H  Z  H  M  P  M  K  O  H  I  C  W
D  D  V  A  S  D  E  F  E  R  E  N  S  H
I  O  A  C  C  I  P  J  V  E  H  Y  D  S
H  M  G  R  R  B  M  N  X  F  G  Y  I  O
C  E  I  O  O  E  Z  Y  T  I  C  S  T  E
R  T  N  S  T  P  S  D  D  N  O  V  A  D
O  R  A  O  U  W  E  B  A  I  J  S  M  Z
T  I  C  M  M  E  Y  N  E  M  D  L  R  V
P  U  A  E  U  D  G  M  I  E  H  I  E  H
Y  M  O  T  C  E  T  A  T  S  O  R  P  B
R  P  E  E  R  M  N  E  G  O  R  T  S  E
C  O  W  P  E  R  S  I  N  X  K  E  A  P
```

Acrosome	Meiosis	Scrotum
Cowpers	Ovaries	Seminiferous
Cryptorchidism	Oviducts	Sperm
Endometrium	Penis	Spermatids
Epididymis	Pregnancy	Vagina
Estrogen	Prostatectomy	Vas deferens

DID YOU KNOW?

The testes produce approximately 50 million sperm per day. Every 2 to 3 months they produce enough cells to populate the entire earth.

There are an estimated 925,000 daily occurrences of STD transmission and 550,000 daily conceptions worldwide.

The United States has one of the highest teen pregnancy rates of all industrialized nations. Rates in France, Germany, and Japan are four times lower.

REPRODUCTIVE SYSTEM

Fill in the crossword puzzle.

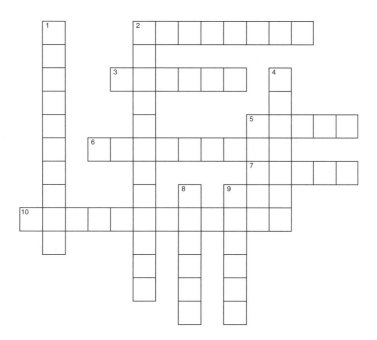

ACROSS

2. Female erectile tissue
3. Colored area around nipple
5. Male reproductive fluid
6. Sex cells
7. External genitalia
10. Male sex hormone

DOWN

1. Failure to have a menstrual period
2. Surgical removal of foreskin
4. Foreskin
8. Menstrual period
9. Essential organs of reproduction

CHECK YOUR KNOWLEDGE

Multiple Choice

Circle the correct answer.

1. What is the membrane that may cover the vaginal opening of the female called?
   A. Hymen
   B. Mons pubis
   C. Labia
   D. Clitoris

2. Which of the following statements is/are true of the menstrual cycle?
   A. Estrogen levels are lowest at the time of ovulation.
   B. Progesterone levels are highest at the time of ovulation.
   C. FSH levels are highest during the proliferation phase.
   D. None of the above are true.

3. A fluid mixture called *semen* could contain which of the following?
   A. Sperm cells
   B. Secretion from the prostate
   C. Secretions from the seminal vesicles
   D. All of the above

4. What is the failure of the testes to descend into the scrotum before birth called?
   A. Cryptococcus
   B. Coccidiomycosis
   C. Cryptorchidism
   D. Cholelithiasis

5. Which of the following is *not* an accessory organ of the female reproductive system?
   A. Breast
   B. Bartholin glands
   C. Ovary
   D. All of the above are accessory organs

6. Which of the following structures can be referred to as *male gonads*?
   A. Testes
   B. Epididymis
   C. Vas deferens
   D. All of the above

7. Sperm cells are suspended outside the body cavity so as to do which of the following?
   A. Protect them from trauma
   B. Keep them at a cooler temperature
   C. Keep them supplied with a greater number of blood vessels
   D. Protect them from infection

8. Surgical removal of the foreskin from the glans penis is called what?
   A. Vasectomy
   B. Sterilization
   C. Circumcision
   D. Ligation

9. What is the colored area around the nipple of the breast called?
   A. Areola
   B. Lactiferous duct
   C. Alveoli
   D. None of the above

10. The female organ that is analogous to the penis in the male is the:
    A. Labia minora
    B. Labia majora.
    C. Vulva.
    D. Clitoris.

Completion

Complete the following statements using the terms listed below. Write the corresponding letter in the answer blank.

A. Clitoris	E. Menses	I. FSH (follicle-stimulating hormone)
B. Endometrium	F. Epididymis	J. Ovulation
C. Ectopic	G. Hysterectomy	K. Scrotum
D. Corpus luteum	H. Prostate	L. Testosterone

11. A pregnancy resulting from the implantation of a fertilized ovum in any location other than the uterus is called _____.

12. Interstitial cells of the testes function to produce _____.

13. The doughnut-shaped accessory organ or gland that surrounds the male urethra is called the _____.

14. Surgical removal of the uterus is called _____.

15. The _____ houses sperm cells as they mature and develop their ability to swim.

16. The skin-covered, external pouch that contains the testes is called the _____.

17. The lining of the uterus is called _____.

18. The hormone progesterone is secreted by a structure called the _____.

19. Fertilization of an egg by a sperm can only occur around the time of _____.

20. From about the first to the seventh day of the menstrual cycle, the anterior pituitary gland secretes _____.

MALE REPRODUCTIVE ORGANS

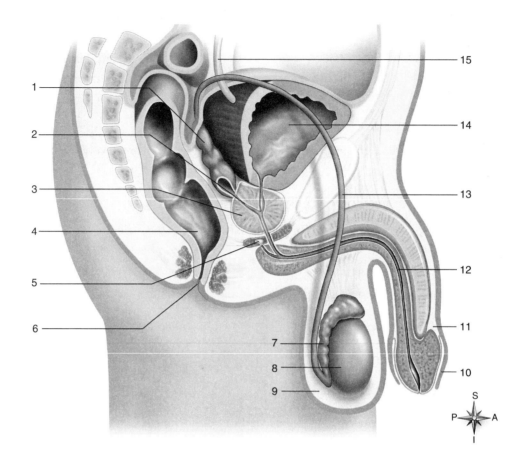

1. _____

2. _____

3. _____

4. _____

5. _____

6. _____

7. _____

8. _____

9. _____

10. _____

11. _____

12. _____

13. _____

14. _____

15. _____

TUBULES OF TESTIS AND EPIDIDYMIS

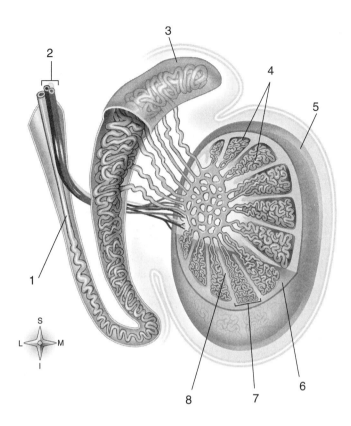

1. _____

2. _____

3. _____

4. _____

5. _____

6. _____

7. _____

8. _____

VULVA

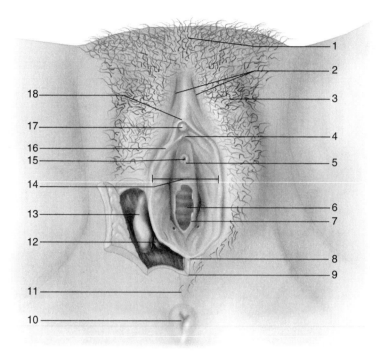

1. _____   10. _____

2. _____   11. _____

3. _____   12. _____

4. _____   13. _____

5. _____   14. _____

6. _____   15. _____

7. _____   16. _____

8. _____   17. _____

9. _____   18. _____

BREAST

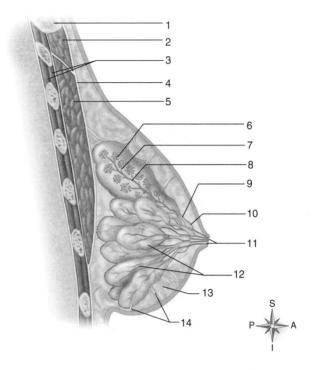

1. _____   8. _____

2. _____   9. _____

3. _____   10. _____

4. _____   11. _____

5. _____   12. _____

6. _____   13. _____

7. _____   14. _____

FEMALE PELVIS

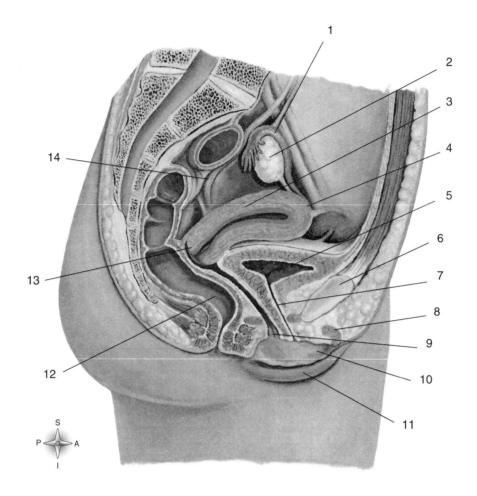

1. _____   8. _____

2. _____   9. _____

3. _____   10. _____

4. _____   11. _____

5. _____   12. _____

6. _____   13. _____

7. _____   14. _____

UTERUS AND ADJACENT STRUCTURES

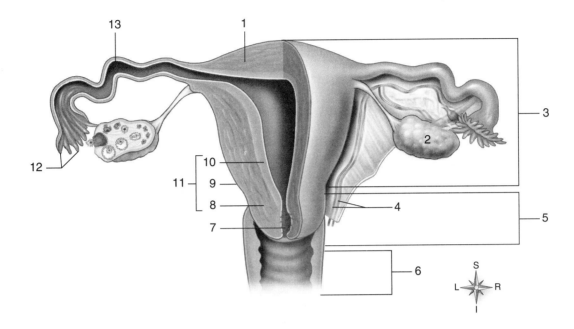

1. _____

2. _____

3. _____

4. _____

5. _____

6. _____

7. _____

8. _____

9. _____

10. _____

11. _____

12. _____

13. _____

Growth and Development

M illions of fragile microscopic sperm swim against numerous obstacles to reach an ovum and create a new life. At birth, the newborn will fill his lungs with air and cry lustily, signaling to the world that he is ready to begin the cycle of life. This cycle will be marked by ongoing changes, periodic physical growth, and continuous development.

This chapter reviews the more significant events that occur in the normal growth and development of an individual from conception to death. Realizing that each person is unique, we nonetheless can discover amid all the complexities of humanity some constants that are understandable and predictable.

Knowledge of human growth and development is essential in understanding the commonalties that influence individuals as they pass through the cycle of life.

TOPICS FOR REVIEW

Before progressing to Chapter 24, you should have an understanding of the concept of development as a biological process. You should familiarize yourself with the major developmental changes from conception through older adulthood. The disorders of pregnancy should be emphasized as you review the chapter. Finally, your study should conclude with a review of the effects of aging on the body systems.

PRENATAL PERIOD
BIRTH OR PARTURITION

Fill in the blanks.

The prenatal stage of development begins at the time of

(1) _____ and continues until

(2) _____. The science of the development of an in-

dividual before birth is called (3) _____. Fertilization

takes place in the outer third of the (4) _____. The

fertilized ovum or (5) _____ begins to divide and in

approximately 3 days forms a solid mass called a

(6) _____. By the time it enters the uterus, it is a hol-

low ball of cells called a (7) _____. As it continues to

develop, it forms a structure with two cavities. The (8) _____

_____ will become a fluid-filled sac for the embryo. The

(9) _____ will develop into an important fetal membrane in the

(10) _____.

Match each description on the left with its corresponding term on the right. Write the letter in the answer blank.

_____ 11. "Within a glass"

_____ 12. Inside germ layer

_____ 13. Before birth

_____ 14. Length of pregnancy

_____ 15. Fiber optic viewing instrument

_____ 16. Process of birth

_____ 17. System used to assess the general condition of a newborn

_____ 18. Study of how the primary germ layers develop into many different kinds of tissues

_____ 19. Term used to describe the developing individual in the first trimester of pregnancy

_____ 20. Monitors progress of developing fetus

A. Laparoscope

B. Gestation

C. Antenatal

D. Histogenesis

E. Apgar score

F. Endoderm

G. In vitro

H. Parturition

I. Embryo

J. Ultrasonogram

▶ *If you had difficulty with this section, review pages 639-650.*

DISORDERS OF PREGNANCY

If the statement is true, write "T" in the answer blank. If the statement is false, correct the statement by circling the incorrect term and writing the correct term in the answer blank.

_____ 21. Many offspring are lost before implantation occurs, often for unknown reasons.

_____ 22. The most common type of ectopic pregnancy is a tubal pregnancy.

_____ 23. If the placenta grows too closely to the cervical opening, a condition called *abruptio placentae* results.

_____ 24. Separation of the placenta from the uterine wall in a pregnancy of 20 weeks or more is known as *placenta previa*.

_____ 25. Toxemia of pregnancy is also known as *puerperal fever*.

_____ 26. After 20 weeks, delivery of a lifeless infant is termed a *miscarriage*.

_____ 27. Acquired birth defects result from agents called *teratogens* that disrupt normal histogenesis and organogenesis.

▶ *If you had difficulty with this section, review pages 649-651.*

POSTNATAL PERIOD

Circle the correct answer.

28. During the postnatal period:
    A. The head becomes proportionately smaller
    B. Thoracic and abdominal contours change from round to elliptical
    C. The legs become proportionately longer
    D. The trunk becomes proportionately shorter
    E. All of the above take place during the postnatal period

29. The period of infancy starts at birth and lasts about:
    A. 4 weeks
    B. 4 months
    C. 10 weeks
    D. 12 months
    E. 18 months

30. The lumbar curvature of the spine appears _____ months after birth.
    A. 1 to 10
    B. 5 to 8
    C. 8 to 12
    D. 11 to 15
    E. 12 to 18

31. During the first 4 months, the birth weight will:
    A. Double
    B. Triple
    C. Quadruple
    D. None of the above

32. At the end of the first year, the weight of the baby will have:
    A. Doubled
    B. Tripled
    C. Quadrupled
    D. None of the above

33. The infant is capable of following a moving object with its eyes at:
    A. 2 days
    B. 2 weeks
    C. 2 months
    D. 4 months
    E. 10 months

34. The infant can lift its head and raise its chest at:
    A. 2 months
    B. 3 months
    C. 4 months
    D. 10 months

35. The infant can crawl at:
    A. 2 months
    B. 3 months
    C. 4 months
    D. 10 months
    E. 12 months

36. The infant can stand alone at:
    A. 2 months
    B. 3 months
    C. 4 months
    D. 10 months
    E. 12 months

37. The permanent teeth, with the exception of the third molar, have all erupted by the age of _____ years.
    A. 6
    B. 8
    C. 12
    D. 14
    E. None of the above

38. Puberty starts at age _____ years in boys.
    A. 10 to 13
    B. 12 to 14
    C. 14 to 16
    D. None of the above

39. Most girls begin breast development at about age:
    A. 8
    B. 9
    C. 10
    D. 11
    E. 12

40. The growth spurt is generally complete by age _____ in males.
    A. 14
    B. 15
    C. 16
    D. 18

41. An average age at which girls begin to menstruate is _____ years.
    A. 10 to 12
    B. 11 to 12
    C. 12 to 13
    D. 13 to 14
    E. 14 to 15

42. The first sign of puberty in boys is:
    A. Facial hair
    B. Increased muscle mass
    C. Pubic hair
    D. Deepening of the voice
    E. Enlargement of the testicles

Match each description on the left with its corresponding term on the right. Write the letter in the answer blank.

_____ 43. Begins at birth and lasts until death

_____ 44. Study of the diagnosis and treatment of disorders of the newborn

_____ 45. Teenage years

_____ 46. From the end of infancy to puberty

_____ 47. Baby teeth

_____ 48. First 4 weeks of infancy

_____ 49. Age at which secondary sexual characteristics occur

_____ 50. Study of aging

_____ 51. Older adulthood

A. Neonatology
B. Neonatal
C. Adolescence
D. Deciduous
E. Puberty
F. Postnatal
G. Gerontology
H. Childhood
I. Senescence

▶ *If you had difficulty with this section, review pages 651-656.*

EFFECTS OF AGING

Fill in the blanks.

52. Old bones develop indistinct and shaggy margins with spurs; a process called
    _____.

53. A degenerative joint disease common in the aged is _____.

54. The number of _____ units in the kidney decreases by almost 50% between the ages of 30 and 75.

55. In old age, respiratory efficiency decreases and a condition known as
    _____ _____ results.

56. Fatty deposits accumulate in blood vessels as we age, and the result is
    _____, which narrows the passageway for the flow of blood.

57. Hardening of the arteries, or _____, occurs during the aging process.

58. Another term for high blood pressure is _____.

59. Hardening of the lens is _____.

60. If the lens becomes cloudy and impairs vision, it is called a _____.

61. _____ causes an increase in the pressure within the eyeball and may result in blindness.

▶ *If you had difficulty with this section, review pages 656-659.*

UNSCRAMBLE THE WORDS

62. **A N N F C Y I**

63. **N A A L T T S O P**

64. **O G S S N E G R A O N E I**

65. **G T E Y Z O**

66. **H D O O L H C I D**

Take the circled letters, unscramble them, and fill in the solution.

The secret to Farmer Brown's prize pumpkin crop.

67.

The secret is in the bag

APPLYING WHAT YOU KNOW

68. Billy's mother told the pediatrician during his 1-year visit that Billy had tripled his birth weight, was crawling actively, and could stand alone. Is Billy's development normal, retarded, or advanced?

69. John is 70 years old. He has always enjoyed food and has had a hearty appetite. Lately, however, he has complained that food "just doesn't taste as good anymore." What might be a possible explanation?

70. Mr. Gaylor has noticed hearing problems but only under certain circumstances. He has difficulty with certain tones, especially high or low tones, but has no problem with everyday conversation. What might be a possible explanation?

71. Mrs. Lowell gave birth to twin girls. The obstetrician, Dr. Sullivan, advised Mr. Lowell that even though the girls looked identical, they were really fraternal twins. How was he able to deduce this?

72. Word Find

Find and circle 13 terms presented in this chapter. Words may be spelled top to bottom, bottom to top, right to left, left to right, or diagonally.

```
F C M P O D N P P A G M J N Z
K E C N E C S E L O D A G G M
I N R B U X T K D A Y Q T F R
L D L T O M S D W A E Z B F E
Z O B A I S P M A L C E E R P
W D I M P L A N T A T I O N L
H E N M K A I T E P D K S X A
W R G A S A R Z R N T Q P Y C
L M Q S I J O O A U B F G T E
R T N T B N G E S T A T I O N
L A T I N E G N O C I T F Z T
D C B T R L A S G C O O R R A
E N O I T I R U T R A P N S B
N V A S N N E G O T A R E T E
```

Adolescence	Implantation	Placenta
Congenital	Laparoscope	Preeclampsia
Endoderm	Mastitis	Progeria
Fertilization	Parturition	Teratogen
Gestation		

DID YOU KNOW?

Brain cells do not regenerate. One beer permanently destroys 10,000 brain cells.

GROWTH/DEVELOPMENT

Fill in the crossword puzzle.

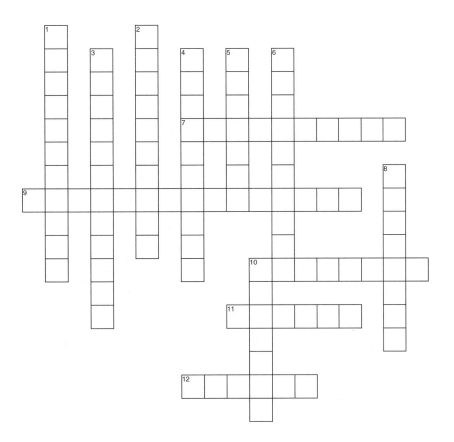

ACROSS

7. Old age
9. Fatty deposit buildup on walls of arteries
10. Cloudy lens
11. Name of zygote after 3 days
12. Fertilized ovum

DOWN

1. Process of birth
2. Science of the development of the individual before birth
3. Study of how germ layers develop into tissues
4. Name of zygote after implantation
5. First 4 weeks of infancy
6. Hardening of the lens
8. Eye disease marked by increased pressure in the eyeball
10. Will develop into a fetal membrane in the placenta

CHECK YOUR KNOWLEDGE

Multiple Choice

Circle the correct answer.

1. When the human embryo is a hollow ball of cells consisting of an outer cell layer and an inner cell mass, what is it called?
   A. Morula
   B. Chorion
   C. Blastocyst
   D. Zygote

2. Degenerative changes in the urinary system that accompany old age include which of the following?
   A. Decreased capacity of the bladder and the inability to empty or void completely
   B. Decrease in the number of nephrons
   C. Less blood flow through the kidneys
   D. All of the above

3. The frontal and maxillary sinuses of the facial region acquire permanent placement or develop fully when the individual is in a stage of development known as which of the following?
   A. Infancy
   B. Childhood
   C. Adolescence
   D. Adulthood

4. The first 4 weeks of human life following birth are referred to as which of the following?
   A. Neonatal
   B. Infancy
   C. Prenatal
   D. Embryonic

5. Any hardening of the arteries is referred to as which of the following?
   A. Angioma
   B. Atherosclerosis
   C. Angina
   D. Arteriosclerosis

6. Which of the following is characteristic of the disorder called *presbyopia*?
   A. It is very characteristic of old age.
   B. It causes farsightedness in some individuals.
   C. It is characterized by the lens in the eye becoming hard and losing its elasticity.
   D. All of the above are true.

7. The three most important "low tech" methods for improving the quality of life as you age are:
   A. Healthy diet, exercise, and stress management
   B. A healthy diet, marriage, and money
   C. A healthy diet, good job, and living in the suburbs
   D. A healthy diet, weight management, and exercise

8. Which of the following events, if any, is *not* characteristic of adolescence?
   A. Bone closure occurs.
   B. Secondary sexual characteristics develop.
   C. Very rapid growth occurs.
   D. All of the above events are characteristic of adolescence.

9. Which of the following events is *not* characteristic of the prenatal period of development?
   A. Blastocyst is formed.
   B. Histogenesis occurs.
   C. Bone closure occurs.
   D. Amniotic cavity is formed.

10. Which of the following structures is derived from ectoderm?
    A. The lining of the lungs
    B. The brain
    C. The kidneys
    D. All of the above

Matching

Match each term in column A with its corresponding definition in column B. (Only one answer is correct for each.)

Column A

_____ 11. Arteriosclerosis

_____ 12. Atherosclerosis

_____ 13. Parturition

_____ 14. Cataract

_____ 15. Adolescence

_____ 16. Amniotic sac

_____ 17. Glaucoma

_____ 18. Senescence

_____ 19. Hypertension

_____ 20. Placenta

Column B

A. High blood pressure

B. Chorion

C. Birth

D. "Bag of waters"

E. Hardening of arteries

F. Degeneration

G. Fat accumulation in arteries

H. Secondary sexual characteristics

I. Clouding of eye lens

J. High eye pressure

FERTILIZATION AND IMPLANTATION

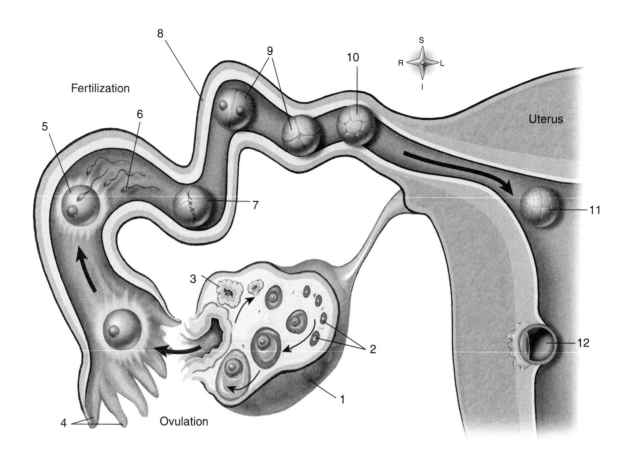

1. _____
2. _____
3. _____
4. _____
5. _____
6. _____
7. _____
8. _____
9. _____
10. _____
11. _____
12. _____

Genetics and Genetic Diseases

L ook around your classroom and you will notice various combinations of hair color, eye color, body size, skin tone, hair texture, gender, etc. Everyone has unique body features and this phenomenon alerts us to the marvel of genetics. Independent units, called *genes*, are responsible for the inheritance of biological traits. Genes determine the structure and function of the human body by producing specific regulatory enzymes. Some genes are dominant and some are recessive. Dominant genes produce traits that appear in the offspring and recessive genes have traits that do not appear in the offspring when they are masked by a dominant gene.

Gene therapy is one of the latest advances of science. This revolutionary branch of medicine combines current technology with genetic research to unlock the secrets of the human body. Daily discoveries in the prevention, diagnosis, treatment, and cure of diseases and disorders are being revealed as a result of genetic therapy. Knowledge of genetics is necessary to understand the basic mechanism by which traits are transmitted from parents to offspring.

TOPICS FOR REVIEW

Your review of this chapter should include an understanding of chromosomes, genes, and gene expression. You should continue your study with a knowledge of common genetic diseases. Finally, your review should conclude with an understanding of the prevention and treatment of genetic diseases.

GENETICS AND HUMAN DISEASE
CHROMOSOMES AND GENES
HUMAN GENOME

Match each term on the left with its corresponding description on the right. Write the letter in the answer blank.

_____ 1. Gene
_____ 2. Chromosome
_____ 3. Gamete
_____ 4. Meiosis
_____ 5. Zygote
_____ 6. Genome
_____ 7. Genomics
_____ 8. Proteomics
_____ 9. Ideogram
_____ 10. Nucleotide base

A. DNA molecule
B. Male or female reproductive cell
C. Special form of nuclear division
D. Formed by union of sperm and ovum at conception
E. Distinct code within a DNA molecule
F. Adenine
G. Entire collection of genetic material in each typical cell
H. Cartoon of a chromosome
I. Analysis of the genome's code
J. Analysis of the proteins encoded by the genome

▷ *If you had difficulty with this section, review pages 665-669.*

GENE EXPRESSION

Fill in the blanks.

After experimentation with pea plants, Mendel discovered that each inherited trait is controlled by two sets of similar (11) _____, one from each parent. He also noted that some genes are (12) _____ and some are (13) _____.
In the example of albinism, a person with the gene combination of Aa is said to be a genetic (14) _____. If two different dominant genes occur together a form of dominance called (15) _____ exists. (16) _____ chromosomes do not have matching structures. If an individual has the sex chromosomes XX, that person will have the sexual characteristics of a (17) _____.
(18) _____ simply means "change." A
(19) _____ _____ is a change in the genetic code.

▷ *If you had difficulty with this section, review pages 669-672.*

GENETIC DISEASES

Match each description on the left with its corresponding term on the right. Write the letter in the answer blank.

_____ 20. Caused by recessive genes in chromosome pair 7

_____ 21. Results in total blindness by age 30

_____ 22. Disease conditions that result from the combined effects of inheritance and environmental factors

_____ 23. Results from a failure to produce the enzyme phenylalanine hydroxylase

_____ 24. Presence of only one autosome instead of a pair

_____ 25. Usually caused by trisomy of chromosome 21

_____ 26. Cystic fibrosis is an example

_____ 27. Results from nondisjunction of chromosomes and typically has the XXY pattern

_____ 28. Term used to describe what happens when a pair of chromosomes fails to separate

_____ 29. Sometimes called *XO syndrome*, it is treated with hormone therapy

A. Single-gene disease

B. Nondisjunction

C. Monosomy

D. Leber hereditary optic neuropathy

E. Cystic fibrosis

F. Phenylketonuria

G. Down syndrome

H. Klinefelter syndrome

I. Turner syndrome

J. Genetic predisposition

 If you had difficulty with this section, review pages 672-676.

PREVENTION AND TREATMENT OF GENETIC DISEASES

Circle the correct answer.

30. A pedigree is a chart that can be used to determine:
    A. Genetic relationships in a family over several generations
    B. The possibility of producing offspring with certain genetic disorders
    C. The possibility of a person developing a genetic disorder late in life
    D. All of the above
    E. None of the above

31. The Punnett square is a grid used to determine:
    A. Genetic disorders
    B. The probability of inheriting genetic traits
    C. Proper gene replacement therapy
    D. The necessity for amniocentesis

32. Some forms of cancer are thought to be caused, at least in part, by abnormal genes called:
    A. Cancercytes
    B. Trisomy
    C. Oncogenes
    D. Autosomes

33. When producing a karyotype, the most common source of cells for the sample is the:
    A. Vagina
    B. Rectum
    C. Lining of the cheek
    D. Throat

34. An ultrasound transducer is used during amniocentesis to:
    A. Create a sharper image
    B. Take measurements during the procedure
    C. Prevent damaging rays during the procedure
    D. Guide the tip of the needle to prevent placental damage

35. Electrophoresis is a process that:
    A. Provides a method for DNA analysis
    B. Means electric separation
    C. Is the basis for DNA fingerprinting
    D. All of the above

36. The use of genetic therapy began in 1990 with a group of young children who had:
    A. AIDS
    B. Adenosine deaminase deficiency
    C. Hemophilia
    D. Cystic fibrosis

If the statement is true, write "T" in the answer blank. If the statement is false, correct the statement by circling the incorrect term and writing the correct term in the answer blank.

_____ 37. Chorionic villus sampling is a procedure in which cells that surround a young embryo are collected through the opening of the cervix.

_____ 38. Karyotyping is the process used for DNA fingerprinting.

_____ 39. In amniocentesis, normal genes are introduced with the hope that they will add to the production of the needed protein.

_____ 40. Deficiency of adenosine deaminase results in severe combined immune deficiency.

_____ 41. One hypothesis that may explain some forms of cancer is known as the *tumor suppressor gene* hypothesis.

▶ *If you had difficulty with this section, review pages 676-681.*

UNSCRAMBLE THE WORDS

42. **R C R R I E A**

43. **Y T S M O I R**

44. **E G N E**

45. **D P E R E G I E**

46. **S O E M C R O S H O M**

Take the circled letters, unscramble them, and fill in the solution.

How Bill made his fortune.

47.

APPLYING WHAT YOU KNOW

48. Steve's mother has a dominant gene for dark skin color. Steve's father has a dominant gene for light skin color. What color will Steve's skin most likely be?

49. Mr. and Mrs. Freund both carry recessive genes for cystic fibrosis. Using your knowledge of the Punnett square, estimate the probability of one of their offspring inheriting this condition.

50. Linda is pregnant and is over 40. She fears her age may predispose her baby to genetic disorders and she has sought the advice of a genetic counselor. What tests might the counselor suggest to alleviate Linda's fears?

51. Punnett Square

Fill in the Punnett square for the following genetic cases:

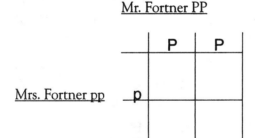

Mr. Fortner PP

Mrs. Fortner pp

Mr. Fortner has two dominant genes for brown eyes and Mrs. Fortner has two recessive genes for blue eyes.

   a. The offspring of Mr. and Mrs. Fortner have a _____ % chance of having brown eyes and a _____ % chance of having blue eyes.
   b. Will Mr. and Mrs. Fortner's offspring be carriers of blue eyes?
   c. If Mr. and Mrs. Fortner's offspring mates with another offspring who is a carrier of blue eyes, what is the probability of the resulting offspring having blue eyes?

Draw your own Punnett square to determine your answer.

Mrs. Harrington Pp

	P	p
P		
p		

Mr. Harrington Pp

Mr. and Mrs. Harrington are both carriers for albinism. Using the Punnett square, determine what percentage of Mr. and Mrs. Harrington's offspring will:

a. Have normal pigmentation _____
b. Be carriers _____
c. Have albinism _____

52. Word Find

Find and circle 14 terms presented in this chapter. Words may be spelled top to bottom, bottom to top, right to left, left to right, or diagonally.

```
N  J  A  T  E  T  O  G  Y  Z  S  F  I  H  Q
M  O  M  D  P  S  I  W  P  L  I  K  Y  E  K
S  M  N  P  E  E  F  Y  A  Z  S  A  X  M  C
F  A  I  D  V  M  M  Z  R  Z  O  R  P  O  L
H  R  O  J  I  O  E  U  E  I  I  Y  D  P  O
I  Q  C  M  S  S  O  L  H  Z  E  O  G  H  X
Y  J  E  O  S  O  J  Z  T  W  M  T  D  I  Q
G  E  N  I  E  M  C  U  E  I  E  Y  X  L  Q
A  O  T  G  C  O  P  K  N  E  J  P  I  I  G
M  P  E  M  E  R  D  A  E  C  P  E  J  A  I
E  D  S  I  R  H  N  C  G  B  T  Z  P  S  Y
T  G  I  D  U  C  G  C  P  X  H  I  F  G  X
E  W  S  R  E  I  R  R  A  C  V  I  O  H  S
S  W  V  B  K  R  C  R  Y  B  V  U  C  N  S
```

Amniocentesis	Gametes	Monosomy
Carrier	Gene therapy	Nondisjunction
Chromosomes	Hemophilia	Recessive
Codominance	Karyotype	Zygote
DNA	Meiosis	

DID YOU KNOW?

Scientists now believe the human body has 50,000 to 100,000 genes packed into just 46 chromosomes.

GENETICS

Fill in the crossword puzzle.

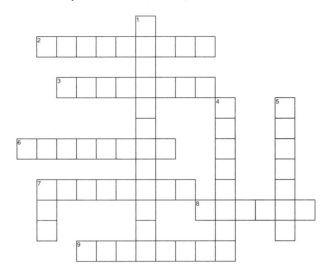

ACROSS

2. Name for the 22 pairs of matched chromosomes
3. Lack of melanin in the skin and eyes
6. Refers to genes that appear in the offspring
7. Chart that illustrates genetic relationships in a family over several generations
8. All genetic material in each cell
9. Scientific study of inheritance

DOWN

1. Trisomy 21 (two words)
4. Agents that cause genetic mutations
5. Triplet of autosomes rather than a pair
7. Excess of phenylketone in the urine (abbreviation)

CHECK YOUR KNOWLEDGE

Multiple Choice

Circle the correct answer.

1. Independent assortment of chromosomes ensures:
   A. Each offspring from a single set of parents is genetically unique
   B. At meiosis, each gamete receives the same number of chromosomes
   C. That the sex chromosomes always match
   D. An equal number of males and females are born

2. Which of the following statements is *not* true of a pedigree?
   A. They are useful to genetic counselors in predicting the possibility of producing offspring with genetic disorders.
   B. They may allow a person to determine his likelihood of developing a genetic disorder later in life.
   C. They indicate the occurrence of those family members affected by a trait, as well as carriers of the trait.
   D. All of the above are true of a pedigree.

3. The genes that cause albinism are:
   A. Codominant
   B. Dominant
   C. Recessive
   D. AA

4. During meiosis, matching pairs of chromosomes line up and exchange genes from their location to the same location on the other side; a process called:
   A. Gene linkage
   B. Crossing-over
   C. Cross-linkage
   D. Genetic variation

5. When a sperm cell unites with an ovum, a _____ is formed.
   A. Zygote
   B. Chromosome
   C. Gamete
   D. None of the above

6. DNA molecules can also be called:
   A. A chromatin strand
   B. A chromosome
   C. A and B
   D. None of the above

7. Nonsexual traits:
   A. Show up more often in females than in males
   B. May be carried on sex chromosomes
   C. Are the result of genetic mutation
   D. All of the above

8. If a person has only X chromosomes, that person is:
   A. Missing essential proteins
   B. Abnormal
   C. Female
   D. Male

9. A karyotype:
   A. Can detect trisomy
   B. Is useful for diagnosing a tubal pregnancy
   C. Is frequently used as a tool in gene augmentation therapy
   D. Can detect the presence of oncogenes

10. Which of the following pairs is mismatched?
    A. SCID—gene therapy
    B. Turner syndrome—trisomy
    C. PKU—recessive
    D. Cystic fibrosis—single-gene disease

Completion

Complete the following statements using the terms listed below. Write the corresponding letter in the answer blank.

A. Cystic fibrosis
B. Males
C. Phenylketonuria
D. Carrier
E. Genome
F. Females

G. Pedigree
H. Oncogenes
I. Karyotype
J. Tay-Sachs disease
K. Amniocentesis
L. Hemophilia

11. Abnormal genes called _____ are believed to be related to cancer.

12. Fetal tissue may be collected by a procedure called _____.

13. An abnormal accumulation of phenylalanine results in _____.

14. The entire collection of genetic material in each cell is called the _____.

15. _____ is caused by recessive genes in chromosome pair seven.

16. A _____ is a chart that illustrates genetic relationships over several generations.

17. A _____ is a person who has a recessive gene that is not expressed.

18. Absence of an essential lipid-producing enzyme may result in the recessive condition _____.

19. _____ is a recessive X-linked disorder.

20. Klinefelter syndrome occurs in _____.

Answers to Exercises

CHAPTER 1
An Introduction to the Structure and Function of the Body

Matching
1. D, p. 4
2. E, p. 6
3. A, p. 6
4. C, p. 6
5. B, p. 6

Matching
6. C, p. 6
7. A, p. 6
8. E, p. 6
9. D, p. 7
10. B, p. 7

Crossword

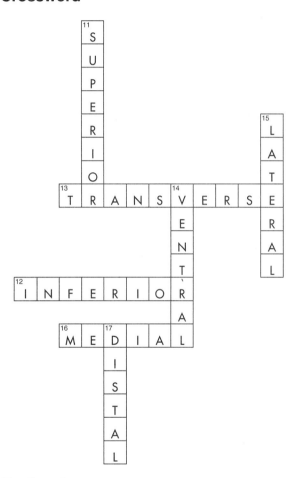

11. Superior
12. Inferior
13. Transverse
14. Ventral
15. Lateral
16. Medial
17. Distal

Did you notice that the answers were arranged as they appear on the human body?

Circle the Correct Answer

18. Inferior, p. 7
19. Anterior, p. 7
20. Lateral, p. 7
21. Proximal, p. 7
22. Superficial, p. 7
23. Equal, p. 8
24. Anterior and posterior, p. 8
25. Upper and lower, p. 8
26. Frontal, p. 8

Select the Correct Term

27. A, p. 10
28. B, p. 10
29. A, p. 10
30. A, p. 10
31. A, p. 10
32. B, p. 10
33. A, p. 10

Circle the One that Does Not Belong

34. Extremities (all others are part of the axial portions)
35. Cephalic (all others are part of the arm)
36. Plantar (all others are part of the face)
37. Carpal (all others are part of the leg or foot)
38. Tarsal (all others are part of the skull)

True or False

39. T
40. F (three stages), p. 11
41. T
42. F (they are not usually dissected), p. 11
43. F (during stage 3), p. 11
44. T

Fill in the Blanks

45. Survival, p. 13
46. Internal environment, p. 13
47. Rise, p. 14
48. Developmental processes, p. 15
49. Aging processes, p. 15
50. Negative, positive, p. 15
51. Stabilizing, p. 15
52. Stimulatory, p. 15

Applying What You Know

53. ① on diagram
54. ② on diagram
55. ③ on diagram

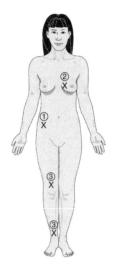

56. **WORD FIND**

Check Your Knowledge

Multiple Choice

1. A, p. 13
2. D, p. 9
3. B, p. 10
4. D, p. 8
5. A, p. 3
6. C, p. 8
7. C, p. 6
8. A, p. 8
9. C, p. 10
10. B, p. 9
11. D, p. 10
12. B, p. 10
13. C, p. 6
14. A, p. 8
15. D, p. 7

16. C, p. 6
17. D, p. 13
18. A, p. 8
19. A, p. 11
20. C, p. 4

Matching

21. F, p. 7
22. B, p. 13
23. J, p. 8
24. G, p. 3
25. H, p. 7
26. C, p. 10
27. D, p. 11
28. I, p. 7
29. A, p. 8
30. E, p. 6

Fill in the blanks

31. Scientific method, p. 16
32. Hypothesis, p. 16
33. Experimentation, p. 16
34. Test group, p. 16
35. Control group, p. 16

Dorsal and Ventral Body Cavities

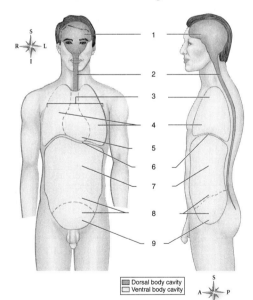

1. Cranial
2. Spinal
3. Thoracic
4. Pleural
5. Mediastinum
6. Diaphragm
7. Abdominal
8. Abdominopelvic
9. Pelvic

Directions and Planes of the Body

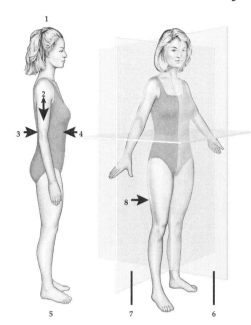

1. Superior
2. Proximal
3. Posterior (dorsal)
4. Anterior (ventral)
5. Inferior
6. Sagittal plane
7. Frontal plane
8. Lateral

Regions of the Abdomen

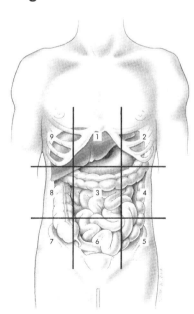

1. Epigastric region
2. Left hypochondriac region
3. Umbilical region
4. Left lumbar region
5. Left iliac (inguinal) region
6. Hypogastric region
7. Right iliac (inguinal) region
8. Right lumbar region
9. Right hypochondriac region

CHAPTER 2
Chemistry of Life

Multiple Choice
1.   C, p. 24
2.   B, p. 24
3.   C, p. 24
4.   A, p. 24
5.   D, p. 24
6.   C, p. 24
7.   A, p. 24

True or False
8.   T, p. 24
9.   F (molecules), p. 24
10. F (uncharged neutrons), p. 24
11. T, p. 24
12. T, p. 24

Multiple Choice
13. C, p. 26
14. B, p. 26
15. A, p. 27
16. B, p. 27
17. A, p. 26
18. C, p. 26

Matching
19. H, p. 27
20. B, p. 27
21. E, p. 27
22. A, p. 28
23. G, p. 28
24. L, p. 28
25. J, p. 28
26. C, p. 28
27. D, p. 29
28. F, p. 29
29. K, p. 30
30. I, p. 30

Circle the Correct Answer
31. A, p. 31
32. B, p. 32
33. D, p. 34
34. B, p. 32
35. C, p. 32
36. A, p. 31
37. A, p. 31
38. B, p. 32
39. C, p. 32
40. D, p. 34

Unscramble the Words
41. Protein

42. Base
43. Alkaline
44. Lipid
45. Salt

Crossword

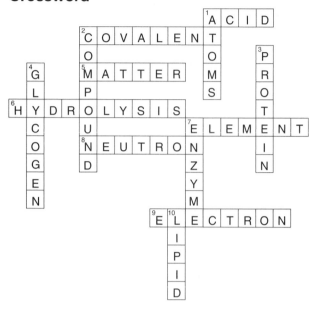

Applying What You Know
46. Some fats can become solid at room temperature, such as the fat in butter and lard.
47. Radioactive isotopes will be used to measure Carol's thyroid activity. A diagnosis of hyperthyroidism or hypothyroidism will be based upon how rapidly or slowly the thyroid absorbs the radioactive iodine and emits radiation.

48. **WORD FIND**

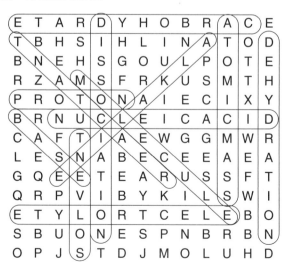

Check Your Knowledge
Fill in the Blanks

1. Biochemistry, p. 23
2. Neutrons, p. 24
3. Higher, p. 24
4. Elements; compounds, p. 24
5. Stable, p. 25
6. Ion, p. 26
7. Inorganic, p. 27
8. Dehydration synthesis, p. 28
9. Chemical equation, p. 28
10. CO_2, p. 29
11. Acids, p. 29
12. Buffers, p. 30
13. Carbohydrate, p. 31
14. Cholesterol, p. 32
15. Structural, p. 32
16. Tertiary protein structure, p. 33
17. Primary protein structure, p. 33
18. Double helix, p. 34
19. Uracil, p. 34
20. Polysaccharides, p. 31

CHAPTER 3
Cells and Tissues

Matching
Group A

1. C, p. 42
2. E, p. 42
3. A, p. 43
4. B, p. 42
5. D, p. 45

Group B

6. D, p. 44
7. E, p. 45
8. A, p. 45
9. B, p. 45
10. C, p. 45

Fill in the Blanks

11. Cholesterol, p. 43
12. Tissue typing, p. 43
13. Cilia, p. 46
14. Endoplasmic reticulum, p. 45
15. Ribosomes, p. 45
16. Mitochondria, p. 45
17. Lysosomes, p. 45
18. Golgi apparatus, p. 45
19. Centrioles, p. 45
20. Chromatin granules, p. 46
21. Rejection reaction, p. 67
22. ELISA, p. 67

Circle the Correct Answer

23. A, p. 48
24. D, p. 48
25. B, p. 48
26. D, p. 49
27. C, p. 49
28. A, p. 49
29. B, p. 49
30. C, p. 50
31. C, p. 50
32. A, p. 51
33. B, p. 50
34. A, p. 50

Circle the One That Does Not Belong

35. Uracil (RNA contains the base uracil, not DNA)
36. RNA (the others are complementary base pairings of DNA)
37. Anaphase (the others refer to genes and heredity)
38. Thymine (the others refer to RNA)
39. Interphase (the others refer to translation)
40. Prophase (the others refer to anaphase)
41. Prophase (the others refer to interphase)
42. Metaphase (the others refer to telophase)
43. Gene (the others refer to stages of cell division)

44. **Fill in the missing areas**

TISSUE	LOCATION	FUNCTION
Epithelial		
1.	1.	1a. Absorption by respiratory gases between alveolar air and blood1b. Diffusion, filtration and osmosis
2.	2a. Surface of lining of mouth and esophagus	2.
	2b. Surface of skin	
3.	3. Surface layer of lining of stomach, intestines, and parts of respiratory tract	3.
4. Stratified transitional	4.	4.
5.	5. Surface of lining of trachea	5.
6.	6.	6. Secretion; absorption
Connective		
1.	1. Between other tissues and organs	1.
2. Adipose	2.	2.
3.	3.	3. Flexible but strong connection
4.	4. Skeleton	4.
5.	5. Part of nasal septum, larynx, rings in trachea and bronchi, disks between vertebrae, external ear	5.
6.	6.	6. Transportation
7. Hematopoietic tissue	7.	7.
Muscle		
1.	1. Muscles that attach to bones, eyeball muscles, upper third of esophagus	1.
2. Cardiac	2.	2.
3.	3. Walls of digestive, respiratory, and genitourinary tracts; walls of blood and large lymphatic vessels; ducts of glands; intrinsic eye muscles; arrector muscles of hair	3.
Nervous		
1. Nervous	1. Brain and spinal cord, nerves	1.

Applying What You Know

45.

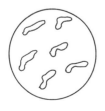

46. Diffusion
47. Absorption of oxygen into Ms. Bence's blood.
48. Merrily may have exceeded the 18 to 24% desirable body fat composition. Fitness depends more on the percentage and ratio of specific tissue types than the overall amount of tissue present.

49. **WORD FIND**

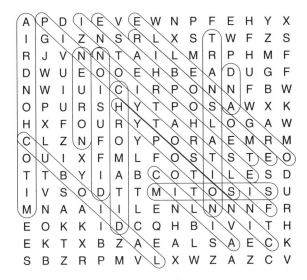

Crossword

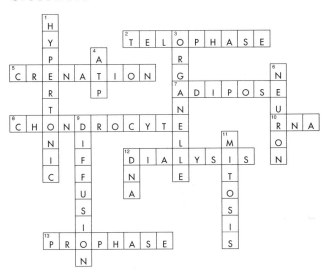

Check Your Knowledge
Multiple Choice

1. A, p. 45
2. B, p. 50
3. B, p. 46
4. A, p. 58
5. C, p. 49
6. A, p. 55
7. A, p. 68
8. B, p. 65
9. C, p. 62
10. D, p. 68

Matching

11. F, p. 66
12. G, p. 43
13. J, p. 69
14. C, p. 52
15. A, p. 57
16. B, p. 54
17. I, p. 48
18. H, p. 62
19. D, p. 45
20. E, p. 61

Cell Structure

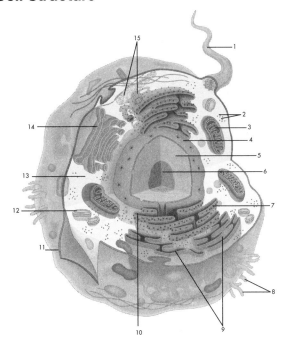

1. Flagellum
2. Free ribosomes
3. Mitochondrion
4. Nuclear envelope
5. Nucleus
6. Nucleolus
7. Ribosomes
8. Cilia
9. Smooth endoplasmic reticulum
10. Rough endoplasmic reticulum
11. Plasma membrane
12. Lysosome
13. Cytoplasm
14. Golgi apparatus
15. Centrioles

Mitosis

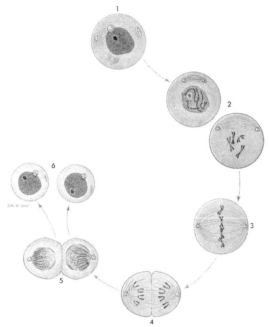

1. Interphase
2. Prophase
3. Metaphase
4. Anaphase
5. Telophase
6. Daughter cells (interphase)

Tissues

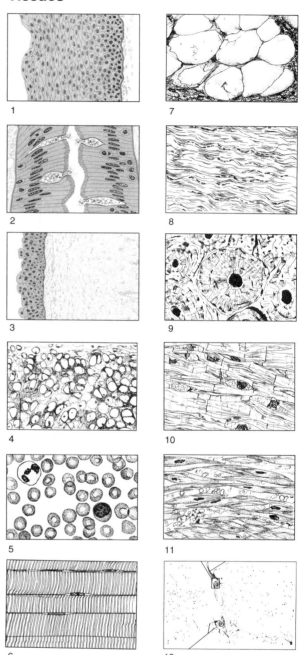

1. Stratified squamous epithelium
2. Simple columnar epithelium
3. Stratified transitional epithelium
4. Cartilage
5. Blood
6. Skeletal muscle
7. Adipose tissue
8. Dense fibrous connective tissue
9. Bone tissue
10. Cardiac muscle
11. Smooth muscle
12. Nervous tissue

CHAPTER 4
Organ Systems of the Body

Matching
Group A

1. A, p. 82
2. E, p. 82
3. D, p. 83
4. B, p. 84
5. C, p. 85

Group B

6. F, p. 85
7. E, p. 86
8. B, p. 88
9. A, p. 88
10. C, p. 87
11. D, p. 90

Circle the One That Does Not Belong

12. Mouth (the others refer to the respiratory system)
13. Rectum (the others refer to the reproductive system)
14. Pancreas (the others refer to the cardiovascular system)
15. Pineal (the others refer to the urinary system)
16. Joints (the others refer to the muscular system)
17. Pituitary (the others refer to the nervous system)
18. Tendons (the others refer to the skeletal system)
19. Appendix (the others refer to the endocrine system)
20. Thymus (the others refer to the integumentary system)
21. Trachea (the others refer to the digestive system)
22. Liver (the others refer to the lymphatic system)

Fill in the Missing Areas

SYSTEM	ORGAN	FUNCTIONS
1..	1.	1. Protection, regulation of body temperature, synthesis of chemicals and hormones, serves as a sense organ
2.	2. Bones, joints	2.
3.	3.	3. Movement, maintains body posture, produces heat
4. Nervous	4.	4.
5.	5. Pituitary, thymus, pineal, adrenal, hypothalamus, thyroid, pancreas, parathyroid, ovaries, testes	5.
6.	6.	6. Transportation, immunity, regulation of body temperature
7.	7. Lymph nodes, lymph vessels, thymus, spleen, tonsils	7.
8. Urinary	8.	8.
9.	9. Mouth, pharynx, esophagus, stomach, small and large intestine, rectum, anal canal, teeth, salivary glands, tongue, liver, gallbladder, pancreas, appendix	9.
10. Respiratory	10.	10.
11.	11a. Gonads—testes and ovaries	11.
	12b. Accessory organs (p. 90), supporting structures (p. 91)	

Fill in the Blanks

24. Nonvital organ, p. 93
25. Cochlear implants, p. 93
26. Dialysis machine, p. 94
27. Left ventricular assist systems (LVAS), p. 94
28. Organ transplantation, p. 94
29. Free-flap surgery, p. 95
30. Rejection, p. 95

Unscramble the Words

31. Heart
32. Pineal
33. Nerve
34. Esophagus
35. Nervous

Applying What You Know

36. (a) Endocrinology (endocrine system)
    (b) Gynecology (reproductive system)
37. The skin protects the underlying tissue against invasion by harmful bacteria. With a large percentage of Brian's skin destroyed, he was vulnerable to bacteria, and so he was placed in the cleanest environment possible—isolation. Jenny is required to wear special attire so that the risk of a visitor bringing bacteria to the patient is reduced.
38. Free-flap surgery may be considered as an option. A breast can be formed from skin and muscle taken from other parts of Sheila's body.

39. **WORD FIND**

Crossword

Check Your Knowledge
Multiple Choice

1. D, p. 88
2. C, pp. 85 and 90
3. C, p. 88
4. B, p. 84
5. D, p. 83
6. A, p. 88
7. B, p. 97
8. A, p. 82
9. A, p. 88
10. C, p. 79

Matching

11. C, p. 82
12. D, p. 85
13. H, p. 86
14. G, p. 90
15. B, p. 88
16. F, p. 88
17. I, p. 91
18. E, p. 87
19. J, p. 84
20. A, p. 85

CHAPTER 5
Mechanisms of Disease

Matching
Group A

1. B, p. 104

2. E, p. 104
3. A, p. 104
4. C, p. 104
5. D, p. 104

Group B

6. C, p. 104
7. A, p. 104
8. D, p. 104
9. B, p. 104
10. E, p. 104

Fill in the Blanks

11. Pathophysiology, p. 106
12. Homeostasis, p. 106
13. Mutated, p. 106
14. Parasite, p. 106
15. Neoplasms, p. 106
16. Self-immunity, p. 107
17. Risk factors, p. 107
18. Centers for Disease Control and Prevention, p. 105
19. Psychogenic, p. 107
20. Secondary, p. 108

Multiple Choice

21. C, p. 108
22. A, p. 111
23. B, p. 109
24. C, p. 111
25. D, p. 112
26. B, p. 112
27. D, p. 114
28. D, p. 115
29. B, p. 116
30. C, p. 116
31. E, p. 116
32. B, p. 117

Circle the Correct Answer

33. Slowly, p. 118
34. Are not, p. 118
35. Papilloma, p. 119
36. Sarcoma, p. 119
37. Anaplasia, p. 120
38. Oncologist, p. 121
39. Biopsy, p. 122
40. Staging, p. 124
41. Appetite, p. 124

Warning Signs of Cancer

42. Sores that do not heal, p. 121
43. Unusual bleeding, p. 121
44. A change in a wart or mole, p. 121
45. A lump or thickening in any tissue, p. 121
46. Persistent hoarseness or cough, p. 121
47. Chronic indigestion, p. 121
48. A change in bowel or bladder function, p. 121
49. Bone pain that wakes the person at night and is located only on one side, p. 121

True or False

50. T
51. F (slowly), p. 126
52. F (white), p. 126
53. T
54. T.
55. T
56. T

Unscramble the Words

57. Fungi
58. Oncogene
59. Edema
60. Spore
61. Grading

Applying What You Know

62. No. Trent most likely has a common cold.
63. Pinworm
64. Disinfection
65. A "gene pool" indicates the "risk" of inheriting a disease-causing gene specific to members of a certain ethnic group. The knowledge of a "gene pool" can alert you to early detection of disease.
66. Bill is considering a "high risk" profession because of the paramedic's frequent exposure to body fluids. Hepatitis B is transmitted by body fluids and, therefore, vaccination is recommended.

67. **WORD FIND**

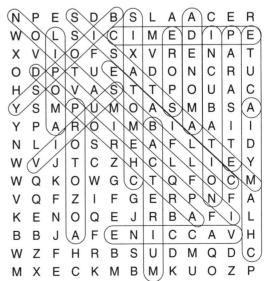

Crossword

```
        ¹N E M ²A T O D E
              D
  ³O N C O G E N E
              N
              O        ⁴M
        ⁵B A C I L L I
              A     ⁶C O C C I
  ⁷V E C T O R     R
              C     O     ⁸P
        ⁹F U N G I  B     U
              N  ¹⁰A M E B A S
              O
      ¹¹E D E M A
              A
```

Check Your Knowledge
Multiple Choice

1. B, p. 104
2. D, p. 104
3. A, p. 118
4. D, p. 104
5. A, p. 113
6. D, p. 104
7. C, p. 105
8. B, p. 124
9. D, p. 108
10. A, p. 114

Matching

11. C, p. 104
12. D, p. 119
13. B, p. 111
14. J, p. 114
15. G, p. 104
16. I, p. 126
17. E, p. 115
18. A, p. 104
19. F, p. 106
20. H, p. 115

Major Groups of Pathogenic Bacteria

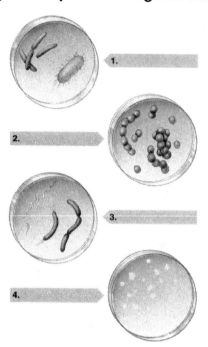

1. Bacilli (rods)
2. Cocci (spheres)
3. Curved rods
4. Small bacteria

Major Groups of Pathogenic Protozoa

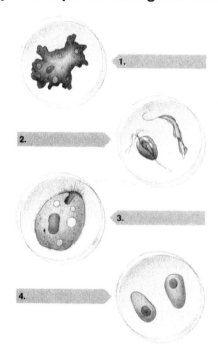

1. Amoebas
2. Flagellates
3. Ciliates
4. Sporozoa

Examples of Pathogenic Animals

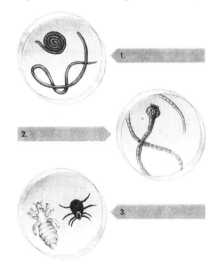

1. Nematodes
2. Platyhelminths
3. Arthropods

Major Groups of Pathogenic Fungi

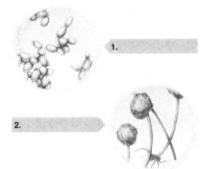

1. Yeasts
2. Molds

CHAPTER 6
The Integumentary System and Body Membranes

Select the Best Answer
1. B, p. 134
2. D, p. 135
3. C, p. 135
4. A, p. 134
5. B, p. 134
6. D, p. 135
7. C, p. 135
8. C, p. 135

Matching
Group A
9. D, p. 133
10. A, p. 136
11. B, p. 136
12. C, p. 136
13. E, p. 136

Group B
14. A, p. 137
15. D, p. 137
16. E, p. 137
17. C, p. 140
18. B, p. 137

Select the Best Answer
19. A, p. 136
20. B, p. 143
21. B, p. 140
22. A, p. 140
23. A, p. 137
24. B, p. 140
25. B, p. 141
26. B, p. 144
27. B, p. 144
28. A, p. 140

Fill in the Blanks
29. Protection, temperature regulation, and sense organ activity, p. 145
30. Melanin, p. 137
31. Lanugo, p. 141
32. Hair papillae, p. 141
33. Alopecia, p. 142
34. Arrector pili, p. 142
35. Strawberry hemangioma, p. 141
36. Eccrine, p. 144
37. Apocrine, p. 144
38. Sebum, p. 144

Circle the Correct Answer
39. Will not, p. 148
40. Will, p. 148
41. Will not, p. 148
42. 11, p. 149
43. Third- , p. 148

Circle the Correct Answer
44. B, p. 146
45. A, p. 147
46. D, p. 150
47. D, p. 150
48. A, p. 149
49. D, p. 150

50. C, p. 150
51. A, p. 152

Unscramble the Words
52. Epidermis
53. Keratin
54. Hair
55. Lanugo
56. Dehydration
57. Third Degree

Applying What You Know
58. 46
59. Pleurisy
60. Sunbathing. Mrs. Collins cannot repair UV damage and thus is very prone to skin cancer.
61. Fingerprints

62. **WORD FIND**

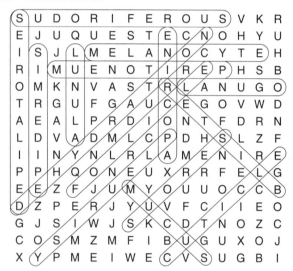

Crossword

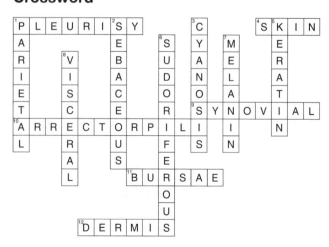

Check Your Knowledge
Multiple Choice
1. A, p. 134
2. B, p. 135
3. A, p. 142
4. D, p. 144
5. B, p. 137
6. D, p. 148
7. B, p. 144
8. B, p. 137
9. C, p. 143
10. B, p. 145

Matching
11. C, p. 137
12. D, p. 134
13. B, p. 143
14. G, p. 144
15. I, p. 137
16. H, p. 141
17. J, p. 143
18. E, p. 135
19. A, p. 140
20. F, p. 144

Completion
21. H, p. 144
22. A, p. 145
23. B, p. 144
24. F, p. 148
25. I, p. 141
26. E, p. 136
27. G, p. 134
28. D, p. 134
29. J, p. 143
30. C, p. 134

Longitudinal Section of the Skin

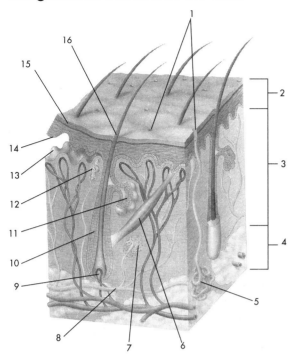

1. Opening of sweat ducts
2. Epidermis
3. Dermis
4. Subcutaneous fatty tissue (hypodermis)
5. Sweat gland
6. Arrector pili muscle
7. Lamellar (Pacini) corpuscle
8. Cutaneous nerve
9. Papilla of hair
10. Hair follicle
11. Sebaceous (oil) gland
12. Tactile (Meissner) corpuscle
13. Dermal papilla
14. Stratum germinativum
15. Stratum corneum
16. Hair shaft

Rule of Nines

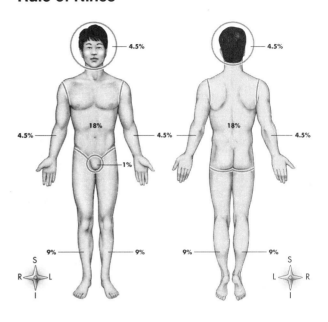

CHAPTER 7
The Skeletal System

Fill in the Blanks
1. Four, p. 164
2. Medullary cavity, p. 164
3. Articular cartilage, p. 165
4. Endosteum, p. 165
5. Hematopoiesis, p. 164
6. Red bone marrow, p. 164
7. Periosteum, p. 165
8. Long, short, flat, and irregular, p. 164
9. Calcium, p. 164
10. Move, p. 164

Matching
Group A

11. D, p. 166
12. B, p. 166
13. E, p. 166
14. A, p. 165
15. C, p. 167

Group B

16. D, p. 167
17. A, p. 167
18. E, p. 167
19. B, p. 167
20. C, p. 166

True or False

21. T
22. F (Epiphyses, not diaphyses), p. 169
23. F (Osteoblasts, not osteoclasts), p. 168
24. T
25. T
26. F (Juvenile, not adult), p. 169
27. F (Diaphysis, not articulation), p. 169
28. T
29. F (Ceases, not begins), p. 169
30. T

Multiple Choice

31. A, p. 170
32. D, p. 172
33. A, p. 176
34. D, p. 178
35. C, p. 180
36. C, p. 182
37. D, p. 180
38. D, p. 180
39. A, p. 182
40. B, p. 174
41. A, p. 176
42. B, p. 180
43. B, p. 178
44. B, p. 180
45. C, p. 180
46. A, p. 182
47. D, p. 172
48. C, p. 176
49. C, p. 172

Circle the One That Does Not Belong

50. Coxal (all others refer to the spine)
51. Axial (all others refer to the appendicular skeleton)
52. Maxilla (all others refer to the cranial bones)
53. Ribs (all others refer to the shoulder girdle)
54. Vomer (all others refer to the bones of the middle ear)
55. Ulna (all others refer to the coxal bone)
56. Ethmoid (all others refer to the hand and wrist)
57. Nasal (all others refer to cranial bones)
58. Anvil (all others refer to the cervical vertebra)

Choose the Correct Answer

59. A, p. 184
60. B, p. 184
61. B, p. 184
62. A, p. 184
63. B, p. 184

Matching

64. C, p. 172
65. G, p. 178
66. J, L, M, and K, p. 182
67. N, p. 182
68. I, p. 180
69. A, p. 172
70. P, p. 182
71. D, B, p. 172
72. F, p. 172
73. H, Q, p. 180
74. O, T, p. 182
75. R, p. 172
76. S, E, p. 172

Circle the Correct Answer

77. Diarthroses, p. 185
78. Synarthrotic, p. 185
79. Diarthrotic, p. 186
80. Ligaments, p. 187
81. Articular cartilage, p. 187
82. Least movable, p. 189
83. Largest, p. 190
84. 2, p. 188
85. Mobility, p. 189
86. Pivot, p. 189

Fill in the Blanks

87. Arthroscopy, p. 199
88. Osteosarcoma, p. 191
89. Osteoporosis, p. 192
90. Osteomalacia, p. 192
91. Paget's disease, p. 193
92. Osteomyelitis, p. 194
93. Simple fractures, p. 196
94. Comminuted fractures, p. 196
95. Osteoarthritis or degenerative joint disease (DJD), p. 196
96. Rheumatoid arthritis, gouty arthritis, and infectious arthritis, p. 197
97. Lyme disease, p. 198

Unscramble the Bones

98. Vertebrae
99. Pubis
100. Scapula
101. Mandible
102. Phalanges
103. Pelvic girdle

Applying What You Know

104. The bones are responsible for the majority of our blood cell formation. Her disease condition might be inhibiting the production of blood cells.
105. Epiphyseal cartilage is present only while a child is still growing. It becomes bone in adult-

hood. It is particularly vulnerable to fractures in childhood and preadolescence.
106. Osteoporosis
107. Slipped or herniated disk

108. **WORD FIND**

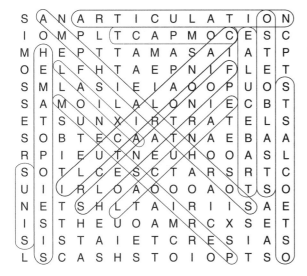

Crossword

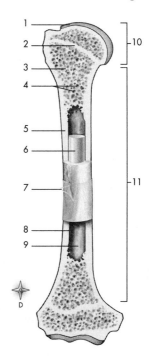

Check Your Knowledge
Multiple Choice

1.   A, p. 177
2.   C, p. 180
3.   A, p. 164
4.   C, p. 184
5.   C, p. 176
6.   D, p. 186
7.   C, p. 170
8.   C, p. 172
9.   D, p. 169
10. A, p. 185

Matching

11. G, p. 187
12. B, p. 166
13. I, p. 185
14. J, p. 172
15. E, p. 182
16. H, p. 167
17. A, p. 166
18. C, p. 172
19. F, p. 182
20. D, p. 164

Longitudinal Section of Long Bone

1.   Articular cartilage
2.   Epiphyseal line
3.   Cancellous (spongy) bone
4.   Red marrow cavities
5.   Compact bone
6.   Yellow marrow
7.   Periosteum
8.   Endosteum
9.   Medullary cavity
10. Epiphysis
11. Diaphysis

Anterior View of Skeleton

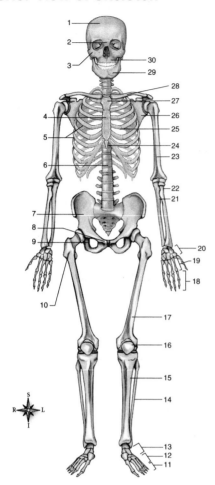

Posterior View of Skeleton

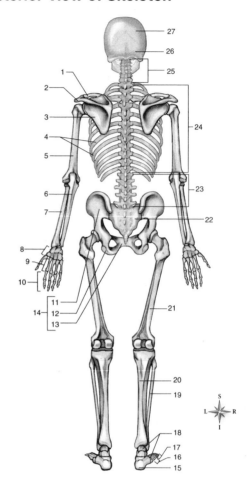

1. Frontal bone
2. Nasal bone
3. Zygomatic bone
4. Sternum
5. Ribs
6. Vertebral column
7. Ilium
8. Pubis
9. Ischium
10. Greater trochanter
11. Phalanges
12. Metatarsals
13. Tarsals
14. Fibula
15. Tibia

16. Patella
17. Femur
18. Phalanges
19. Metacarpals
20. Carpals
21. Ulna
22. Radius
23. Humerus
24. Xiphoid process
25. Costal cartilage
26. Scapula
27. Manubrium
28. Clavicle
29. Mandible
30. Maxilla

1. Clavicle
2. Acromion process
3. Scapula
4. Ribs
5. Humerus
6. Ulna
7. Radius
8. Carpals
9. Metacarpals
10. Phalanges
11. Ilium
12. Ischium
13. Pubis
14. Coxal (hip) bone

15. Calcaneus (a tar-
     sal bone)
16. Metatarsal bones
17. Phalanges
18. Tarsals
19. Fibula
20. Tibia
21. Femur
22. Sacrum
23. Lumbar vertebrae
24. Thoracic vertebrae
25. Cervical vertebrae
26. Occipital bone
27. Parietal bone

Skull Viewed from the Right Side

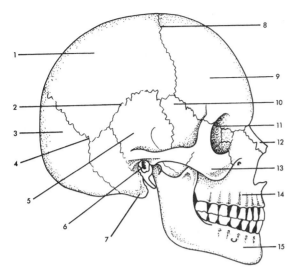

1. Parietal bone
2. Squamous suture
3. Occipital bone
4. Lambdoidal suture
5. Temporal bone
6. External auditory canal
7. Mastoid process
8. Coronal suture
9. Frontal bone
10. Sphenoid bone
11. Ethmoid bone
12. Nasal bone
13. Zygomatic bone
14. Maxilla
15. Mandible

Skull Viewed from the Front

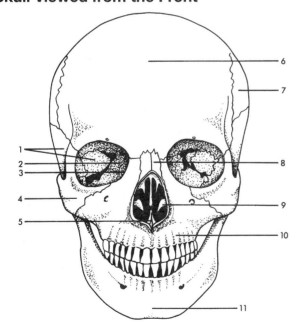

1. Sphenoid bone
2. Ethmoid bone
3. Lacrimal bone
4. Zygomatic bone
5. Vomer
6. Frontal bone
7. Parietal bone
8. Nasal bone
9. Inferior concha
10. Maxilla
11. Mandible

Diarthrotic Joint

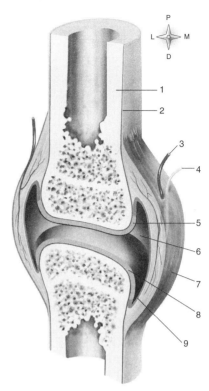

1. Bone
2. Periosteum
3. Blood vessel
4. Nerve
5. Articular cartilage
6. Joint cavity
7. Joint capsule
8. Articular cartilage
9. Synovial membrane

CHAPTER 8
The Muscular System

Select the Correct Term
1. A, p. 208
2. B, p. 208
3. C, p. 208
4. C, p. 208
5. A, p. 208
6. B, p. 208
7. C, (may also be B), p. 208 and Chapter 3
8. A, p. 208
9. C, p. 208
10. C, p. 208

Matching
Group A

11. D, p. 208

12. B, p. 208
13. A, p. 208
14. E, p. 208
15. C, p. 208

Group B

16. E, p. 209
17. C, p. 209
18. B, p. 209
19. A, p. 209
20. D, p. 209

Fill in the Blanks

21. Pulling, p. 211
22. Insertion, p. 211
23. Insertion, origin, p. 211
24. Prime mover, p. 211
25. Antagonists, p. 211
26. Synergist, p. 211
27. Tonic contraction, p. 211
28. Muscle tone, p. 211
29. Hypothermia, p. 211
30. ATP, p. 211

True or False

31. F (Neuromuscular junction), p. 213
32. T
33. T
34. F (Oxygen debt), p. 212
35. F ("All or none"), p. 214
36. F (Lactic acid), p. 212
37. T
38. T
39. F (Skeletal muscles), p. 213
40. T

Multiple Choice

41. A, p. 214
42. B, p. 214
43. B, p. 214
44. C, p. 215
45. D, p. 214
46. A, p. 214
47. B, p. 214
48. C, p. 214
49. B, p. 215
50. D, p. 215

Matching

51. C, p. 217
52. F, p. 217; A and D, p. 223
53. F, p. 217 and B, p. 223
54. A, p. 223
55. C, p. 223
56. B, p. 217 and F, p. 223

57. A, p. 223
58. A and D, p. 223
59. B, p. 223
60. B, p. 223
61. A and E, p. 217
62. B, p. 217
63. D, p. 217

Multiple Choice

64. A, p. 222
65. D, p. 222
66. C, p. 222
67. A, p. 222
68. D, p. 222
69. C, p. 222

Circle the Correct Answer

70. Myalgia, p. 224
71. Myoglobin, p. 224
72. Poliomyelitis, p. 224
73. Muscular dystrophy, p. 225
74. Myasthenia gravis, p. 225

Applying What You Know

75. Bursitis
76. Deltoid area
77. Tendon

78. **WORD FIND**

Crossword

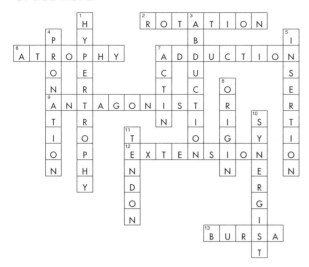

Check Your Knowledge
Multiple Choice

1. D, p. 213
2. A, p. 222
3. C, p. 210
4. B, p. 217
5. A, p. 214
6. B, p. 212
7. D, p. 214
8. A, p. 215
9. A, p. 214
10. C, p. 211

True or False

11. T, p. 222
12. T, p. 214
13. F (Pronation), p. 222
14. F (Hypertrophy), p. 215
15. T, p. 214
16. T, p. 211
17. T, p. 211
18. F (Hypothermia), p. 215
19. T, p. 214
20. F (Flexion), p. 222

Muscles—Anterior View

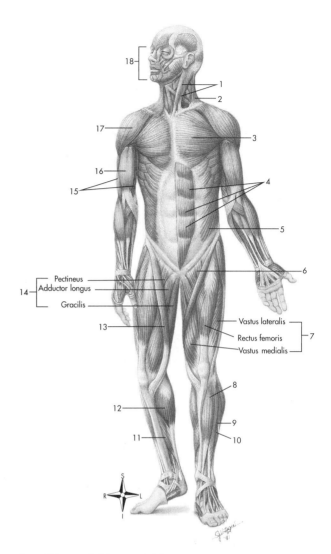

1. Sternocleidomastoid
2. Trapezius
3. Pectoralis major
4. Rectus abdominis
5. External abdominal oblique
6. Iliopsoas
7. Quadriceps group
8. Tibialis anterior
9. Peroneus longus
10. Peroneus brevis
11. Soleus
12. Gastrocnemius
13. Sartorius
14. Adductor group
15. Brachialis
16. Biceps brachii
17. Deltoid
18. Facial muscles

Muscles—Posterior View

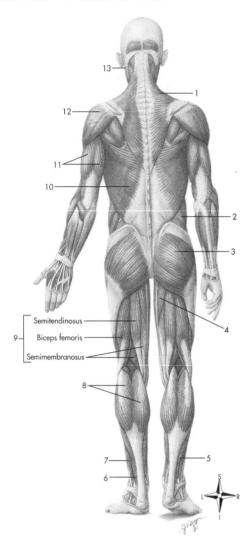

Labels on figure:
13
12
1
11
10
2
3
4
Semitendinosus
Biceps femoris
9
Semimembranosus
8
7 5
6
S
L R
I

1. Trapezius
2. External abdominal oblique
3. Gluteus maximus
4. Adductor magnus
5. Soleus
6. Peroneus brevis
7. Peroneus longus
8. Gastrocnemius
9. Hamstring group
10. Latissimus dorsi
11. Triceps brachii
12. Deltoid
13. Sternocleidomastoid

CHAPTER 9
The Nervous System

Matching
Group A

1. B, p. 236
2. C, p. 236
3. D, p. 236
4. A, p. 236

Group B

5. B, p. 236
6. D, p. 237
7. C, p. 236
8. A, p. 237
9. F, p. 240
10. E, p. 240

Select the Best Choice

11. A, p. 236
12. B, p. 237
13. B, p. 238
14. A, p. 236
15. A, p. 236
16. B, p. 238
17. B, p. 238
18. A, p. 236
19. B, p. 238
20. A, p. 239

Fill in the Blanks

21. Two-neuron arc, p. 241
22. Sensory neurons, interneurons, and motor neurons, p. 241
23. Receptors, p. 241
24. Synapse, p. 241
25. Reflex, p. 241
26. Withdrawal reflex, p. 242
27. Ganglion, p. 241
28. Interneurons, p. 242
29. "Knee jerk," p. 242
30. Gray matter, p. 241

Circle the Correct Answer

31. Do not, p. 242
32. Increases, p. 244
33. Excess, p. 242
34. Postsynaptic, p. 244
35. Presynaptic, p. 244
36. Neurotransmitter, p. 244
37. Communicate, p. 244
38. Specifically, p. 244
39. Sleep, p. 245
40. Pain, p. 245

Multiple Choice

41. E, p. 247
42. D, p. 247
43. A, p. 247
44. E, p. 248
45. E, p. 248
46. D, p. 249
47. B, p. 249
48. E, p. 249
49. B, p. 251
50. D, p. 251
51. D, p. 247
52. B, p. 249
53. A, p. 251
54. D, p. 249
55. C, p. 249

Select the Best Choice

56. H, p. 251
57. D, p. 251
58. E, p. 251
59. C, p. 254
60. J, p. 254
61. A, p. 254
62. B, p. 254
63. F, p. 254
64. I, p. 252
65. G, p. 252

True or False

66. F (17 to 18 inches), p. 255
67. F (Bottom of the first lumbar vertebra), p. 255
68. F (Lumbar punctures), p. 260
69. F (Spinal tracts), p. 256
70. T
71. F (One general function), p. 256
72. F (Anesthesia), p. 257

Circle the One That Does Not Belong

73. Ventricles (all others refer to meninges)
74. CSF (all others refer to the arachnoid)
75. Pia mater (all others refer to the cerebrospinal fluid)
76. Choroid plexus (all others refer to the dura mater)
77. Brain tumor (all others refer to a lumbar puncture)

Cranial Nerves

78. Fill in the missing areas on the chart below.

Nerve		Conduct Impulses	Function
I	Olfactory		
II			Vision
III		From brain to eye muscles	
IV	Trochlear		
V			Sensations of face, scalp, and teeth, chewing movements
VI		From brain to external eye muscles	
VII			Sense of taste; Contraction of muscles of facial expression
VIII	Vestibulocochlear		
IX		From throat and taste buds of tongue to brain; also from brain to throat muscles and salivary glands	
X	Vagus		
XI			Shoulder movements; turning movements of head
XII	Hypoglossal		

Select the Best Choice
79. A, p. 260
80. B, p. 262
81. A, p. 260
82. B, p. 263
83. B, p. 261
84. A, p. 260
85. B, p. 261
86. B, p. 261

Matching
87. D, p. 264
88. E, p. 264
89. F, p. 264
90. B, p. 264
91. A, p. 264
92. C, p. 264

Multiple Choice
93. C, p. 267
94. B, p. 267
95. B, p. 267
96. D, p. 267
97. A, p. 267
98. A, p. 268

Choose the Correct Answer
99. B, p. 267
100. A, p. 267
101. A, p. 267
102. B, p. 267
103. A, p. 267
104. B, p. 267
105. A, p. 267
106. A, p. 267
107. B, p. 267
108. B, p. 267

Fill in the Blanks
109. Acetylcholine, p. 268
110. Adrenergic fibers, p. 268
111. Cholinergic fibers, p. 268
112. Homeostasis, p. 268
113. Heart rate, p. 268
114. Decreased, p. 268
115. Neuroblastoma, p. 268

Unscramble the Words
116. Neurons
117. Synapse
118. Autonomic
119. Smooth muscle
120. Sympathetic

Applying What You Know
121. Right

122. Hydrocephalus
123. Sympathetic
124. Parasympathetic
125. Sympathetic. No, the digestive process is not active during sympathetic control. Bill may experience nausea, vomiting, or discomfort because of this factor. See p. 267.

126. **WORD FIND**

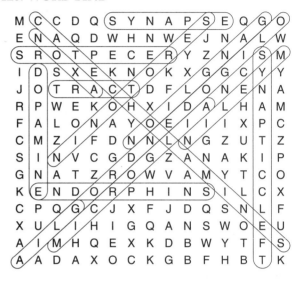

Crossword

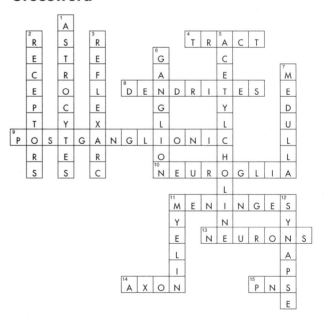

Check Your Knowledge
Multiple Choice

1.   D, p. 236
2.   B, p. 257
3.   A, p. 257
4.   B, p. 247
5.   A, p. 267

6. D, p. 268
7. D, p. 237
8. C, p. 244
9. C, p. 256
10. D, p. 264

Matching

11. C, p. 256
12. A, p. 236
13. J, p. 247
14. H, p. 244
15. B, p. 237
16. I, p. 262
17. F, p. 237
18. E, p. 247
19. D, p. 260
20. G, p. 269

Structure of a Neuron

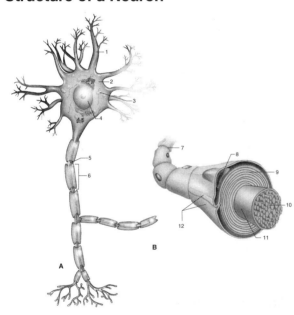

1. Dendrites
2. Cell body
3. Mitochondrion
4. Nucleus
5. Axon
6. Schwann cell
7. Node of Ranvier
8. Nucleus of Schwann cell
9. Myelin sheath
10. Axon
11. Cell membrane of axon
12. Neurilemma (sheath of Schwann cell)

Cranial Nerves

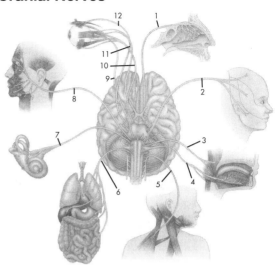

1. Olfactory nerve (I)
2. Trigeminal nerve (V)
3. Glossopharyngeal nerve (IX)
4. Hypoglossal nerve (XII)
5. Accessory nerve (XI)
6. Vagus nerve (X)
7. Vestibulocochlear nerve (VIII)
8. Facial nerve (VII)
9. Abducens nerve (VI)
10. Oculomotor nerve (III)
11. Optic nerve (II)
12. Trochlear nerve (IV)

Sagittal Section of the Central Nervous System

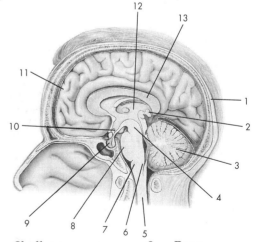

1. Skull
2. Pineal gland
3. Cerebellum
4. Midbrain
5. Spinal cord
6. Medulla
7. Reticular formation
8. Pons
9. Pituitary gland
10. Hypothalamus
11. Cerebral cortex
12. Thalamus
13. Corpus callosum

The Cerebrum

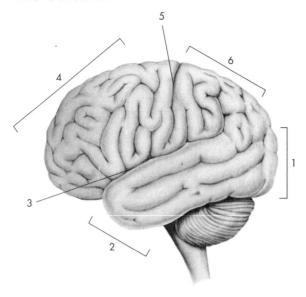

1. Occipital lobe
2. Temporal lobe
3. Lateral fissure
4. Frontal lobe
5. Central Sulcus
6. Parietal lobe

Neuron Pathways

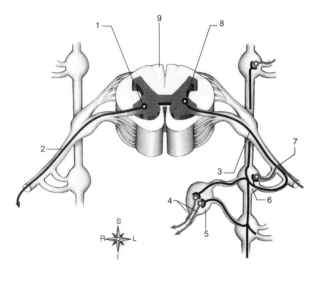

1. Cell body of somatic motor neuron
2. Axon of somatic motor neuron
3. Axon of preganglionic sympathetic neuron
4. Postganglionic neuron's axon
5. Collateral ganglion
6. Sympathetic ganglion
7. Postganglionic neuron's axon
8. Cell body of preganglionic neuron
9. Spinal cord

CHAPTER 10
The Senses

Matching
1. D, p. 282
2. B, p. 282
3. A, p. 283
4. E, p. 282
5. C, p. 283

Multiple Choice
6. C, p. 284
7. E, p. 284
8. B, p. 284
9. C, p. 285
10. E, p. 285
11. D, p. 286
12. A, p. 286
13. B, p. 286
14. C, p. 287
15. B, p. 287
16. D, p. 286
17. A, p. 287
18. D, p. 287

Select the Best Answer
19. C, p. 288
20. E, p. 289
21. F, p. 289
22. A, p. 290
23. J, p. 286
24. B, p. 291
25. H, p. 288
26. G, p. 291
27. I, p. 294
28. D, p. 287

Select the Best Answer
29. B, p. 296
30. C, p. 296
31. B, p. 296
32. A, p. 295
33. C, p. 297
34. A, p. 294
35. C, p. 297
36. B, p. 296
37. A, p. 295
38. C, p. 297

Fill in the Blanks
39. Auricle; external acoustic canal, p. 294
40. Eardrum, p. 295
41. Ossicles, p. 296
42. Oval window, p. 296
43. Otitis media, p. 296

44. Vestibule, p. 296
45. Mechanoreceptors, p. 297
46. Crista ampullaris, p. 297

Select the Best Answer

47. C, p. 299
48. A, p. 299
49. D, p. 299
50. E, p. 299
51. B, p. 299
52. F, p. 299

Circle the Correct Answer

53. Papillae, p. 300
54. Cranial, p. 300
55. Mucus, p. 300
56. Memory, p. 301
57. Chemoreceptors, p. 300

Unscramble the Words

58. Auricle
59. Sclera
60. Papilla
61. Conjunctiva
62. Pupils

Applying What You Know

63. External otitis
64. Cataracts
65. The eustachian tube connects the throat to the middle ear and provides a perfect pathway for the spread of infection.
66. Olfactory

67. **WORD FIND**

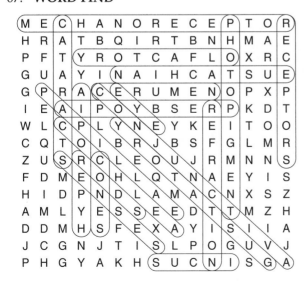

Crossword

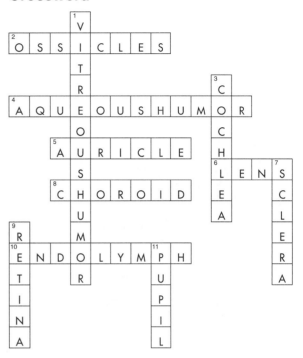

Check Your Knowledge
Multiple Choice

1. A, p. 297
2. B, p. 297
3. A, p. 300
4. C, p. 293
5. B, p. 284
6. B, p. 282
7. D, p. 286
8. B, p. 285
9. D, p. 300
10. A, p. 294

True or False

11. T, p. 295
12. F (Aqueous humor), p. 287
13. T, p. 286
14. F (malleus, incus and stapes), p. 296
15. T, p. 288
16. T, p. 285
17. T, p. 286
18. T, p. 284
19. T, p. 300
20. T, p. 296

Eye

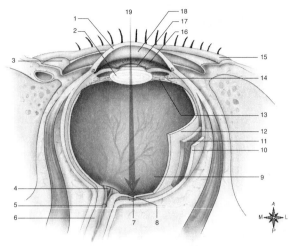

1. Cornea
2. Lens
3. Lacrimal caruncle
4. Optic disc
5. Central artery and vein
6. Optic nerve
7. Fovea
8. Macula
9. Posterior chamber (contains vitreous humor)
10. Sclera
11. Choroid
12. Retina
13. Suspensory ligament
14. Ciliary muscle
15. Lower lid
16. Iris
17. Pupil
18. Anterior chamber (contains aqueous humor)
19. Visual (optic) axis

Ear

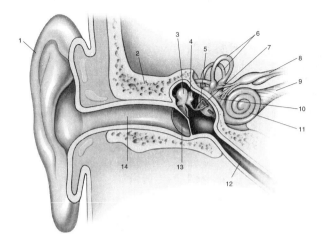

1. Auricle (pinna)
2. Temporal bone
3. Malleus
4. Incus
5. Stapes
6. Semicircular canals
7. Oval window
8. Vestibular nerve
9. Cochlear nerve
10. Vestibule
11. Cochlea
12. Auditory tube
13. Tympanic membrane
14. External auditory meatus

CHAPTER 11
The Endocrine System

Matching
Group A

1. D, p. 310
2. C, p. 310
3. E, p. 310
4. A, p. 310
5. B, p. 310

Group B

6. E, p. 314
7. C, p. 316
8. A, p. 316
9. D, p. 310
10. B, p. 310

Fill in the Blanks

11. Second messenger, p. 310
12. Protein, p. 310

13. First messenger, p. 310
14. Target organs, p. 310
15. Cyclic AMP, p. 311
16. Target cells, p. 311
17. Steroid abuse, p. 314

Multiple Choice
18. B, p. 317
19. E, p. 312
20. D, p. 312
21. D, p. 317
22. A, p. 317
23. C, p. 318
24. C, p. 319
25. B, p. 317
26. A, p. 317
27. A, p. 317
28. D, p. 318
29. B, p. 318
30. A, p. 319
31. C, p. 319
32. C, p. 320

Select the Best Answer
33. A, p. 317
34. B, p. 317
35. B, p. 319
36. C, p. 320
37. A, p. 317
38. C, p. 320
39. A, p. 317
40. A, p. 317
41. A, p. 317
42. C, p. 320

Circle the Correct Answer
43. Below, p. 320
44. Calcitonin, p. 320
45. Iodine, p. 320
46. Do not, p. 320
47. Thyroid, p. 320
48. Decreases, p. 320
49. Hypothyroidism, p. 322
50. Cretinism, p. 322
51. PTH, p. 323
52. Increase, p. 323

Fill in the Blanks
53. Adrenal cortex; adrenal medulla, p. 323
54. Corticoids, p. 324
55. Mineralocorticoids, p. 324
56. Glucocorticoids, p. 324
57. Sex hormones, p. 324
58. Gluconeogenesis, p. 324
59. Blood pressure, p. 325

60. Epinephrine; norepinephrine, p. 326
61. Stress, p. 326
62. Virilizing, p. 327

Select the Best Response
63. A, p. 327
64. A, p. 325
65. B, p. 313
66. A, p. 327
67. B, p. 326
68. A, p. 324
69. A, p. 327

Circle the Term That Does Not Belong
70. Beta cells (all others refer to glucagon)
71. Glucagon (all others refer to insulin)
72. Thymosin (all others refer to female sex glands)
73. Chorion (all others refer to male sex glands)
74. Aldosterone (all others refer to the thymus gland)
75. ACTH (all others refer to the placenta)
76. Semen (all others refer to the pineal gland)

Matching
Group A
77. E, p. 328
78. C, p. 328
79. B, p. 330
80. D, p. 331
81. A, p. 330

Group B
82. E, p. 331
83. A, p. 331
84. B, p. 331
85. C, p. 331
86. D, p. 331

Unscramble the Words
87. Corticoids
88. Diuresis
89. Glucocorticoids
90. Steroids
91. Stress

Applying What You Know
92. She was pregnant.
93. The inner zone reticularis of the adrenal cortex
94. Oxytocin

95.   **WORD FIND**

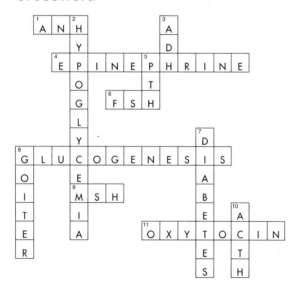

Crossword

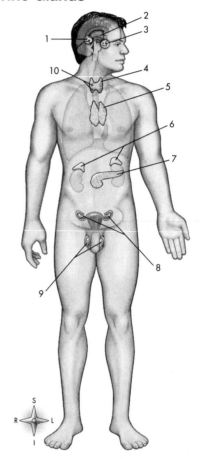

Check Your Knowledge
Multiple Choice

1.   A, p. 324
2.   C, p. 319
3.   D, p. 322
4.   B, p. 317
5.   D, p. 312
6.   D, p. 318
7.   B, p. 331
8.   D, p. 325
9.   D, p. 328
10.   B, p. 316

Matching

11.   J, p. 322
12.   G, p. 317

13.   H, p. 328
14.   I, p. 318
15.   B, p. 319
16.   F, p. 331
17.   A, p. 327
18.   D, p. 319
19.   E, p. 318
20.   C, p. 321

Endocrine Glands

1.   Pineal
2.   Hypothalamus
3.   Pituitary
4.   Thyroid
5.   Thymus
6.   Adrenals
7.   Pancreas (islets)
8.   Ovaries (female)
9.   Testes (male)
10.   Parathyroids

CHAPTER 12
Blood

Multiple Choice
1. E, p. 342
2. D, p. 342
3. D, p. 342
4. A, p. 343
5. D, p. 343

Fill in the Blank Areas
6.

Blood Type	Antigen Present in RBC	Antibody Present in Plasma
A	A	Anti-B
B	B	Anti-A
AB	A, B	None
O	None	Anti-A, Anti-B

Fill in the Blanks
7. Antigen, p. 344
8. Antibody, p. 344
9. Agglutinate, p. 344
10. Erythroblastosis fetalis, p. 345
11. Rhesus monkey, p. 345
12. Type O, p. 345
13. Type AB, p. 345

Multiple Choice
14. B, p. 346
15. C, p. 346
16. A, p. 352
17. B, p. 350
18. D, p. 346.
19. C, p. 351
20. D, p. 348
21. A, p. 353
22. B, p. 350
23. B, p. 349
24. B, p. 346
25. E, p. 348
26. B, p. 347
27. C, p. 347
28. D, p. 347
29. D, p. 350
30. D, p. 350
31. B, p. 356
32. D, p. 349
33. B, p. 356
34. C, p. 357
35. B, p. 357
36. A, p. 361

37. E, p. 362
38. B, p. 352
39. C, p. 353
40. A, p. 362
41. C, p. 356

Applying What You Know
42. No. If Mrs. Florez were a negative Rh factor and her husband were a positive Rh factor, it would set up the strong possibility of erythroblastosis fetalis.
43. Both procedures assist the clotting process.
44. Anemia

45. **WORD FIND**

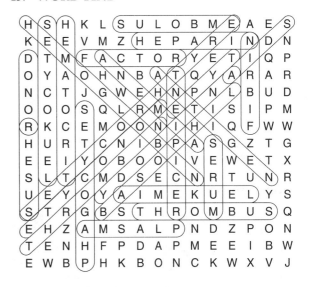

Crossword

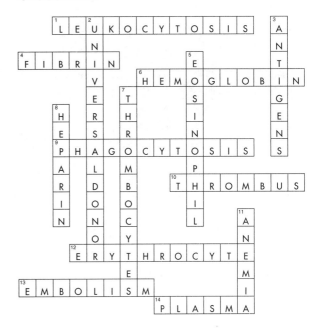

Check Your Knowledge
Multiple Choice

1. B, p. 358
2. B, p. 351
3. A, p. 348
4. A, p. 346
5. D, p. 342
6. A, p. 356
7. A, p. 362
8. D, p. 345
9. C, p. 348
10. B, p. 360

Matching

11. D, p. 357
12. F, p. 351
13. H, p. 345
14. A, p. 356
15. G, p. 358
16. C, p. 360
17. B, p. 345
18. E, p. 345
19. I, p. 347
20. J, p. 356

Human Blood Cells

BODY CELL		FUNCTION
Erythrocyte		Oxygen and carbon dioxide transport
Neutrophil		Immune defense (phagocytosis)
Eosinophil		Defense against parasites
Basophil		Inflammatory response and heparin secretion
B lymphocyte		Antibody production (precursor of plasma cells)
T lymphocyte		Cellular immune response
Monocyte		Immune defenses (phagocytosis)
Thrombocyte		Blood clotting

Blood Typing

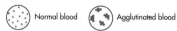

Recipient's blood		Reactions with donor's blood			
RBC antigens	Plasma antibodies	Donor type O	Donor type A	Donor type B	Donor type AB
None (Type O)	Anti-A Anti-B				
A (Type A)	Anti-B				
B (Type B)	Anti-A				
AB (Type AB)	(none)				

 Normal blood   Agglutinated blood

CHAPTER 13
The Heart and Heart Disease

Fill in the Blanks

1. Circulatory system, p. 373
2. Apex, p. 375
3. Interatrial septum, p. 376
4. Atria, p. 376
5. Ventricles, p. 376
6. Myocardium, p. 376
7. Endocarditis, p. 376
8. Bicuspid or mitral and tricuspid, p. 378
9. Visceral pericardium or epicardium, p. 376
10. Parietal pericardium, p. 376
11. Pericarditis, p. 376
12. Semilunar valves, p. 378
13. Mitral valve prolapse, p. 378
14. Rheumatic heart disease, p. 378

Select the Best Answer

15. F, p. 380
16. C, p. 381
17. D, p. 381
18. A, p. 379
19. B, p. 380
20. G, p. 381
21. E, p. 381
22. H, p. 381
23. J, p. 380
24. I, p. 381

Circle the Correct Answer

25. B, p. 382
26. C p. 382
27. A, p. 382
28. C, p. 386
29. A, p. 384
30. D, p. 384

31. C, p. 386
32. A, p. 387
33. B, p. 388
34. C, p. 388
35. A, p. 387
36. D, p. 387

Unscramble the Words
37. Systemic
38. Mitral
39. Heart
40. Thrombus
41. Rhythm

Applying What You Know
42. Coronary bypass surgery
43. Artificial pacemaker
44. The endocardial lining can become rough and abrasive to red blood cells passing over its surface. As a result, a fatal blood clot may be formed.
45. 3   Tricuspid valve
    6   Pulmonary arteries
    9   Bicuspid valve
    1   Vena cavae
    4   Right ventricle
    12   Aorta
    7   Pulmonary veins
    5   Pulmonary semilunar valve
    10   Left ventricle
    2   Right atrium
    8   Left atrium
    11   Aortic semilunar valve

46. **WORD FIND**

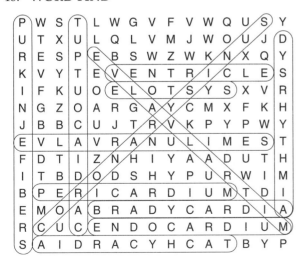

Crossword

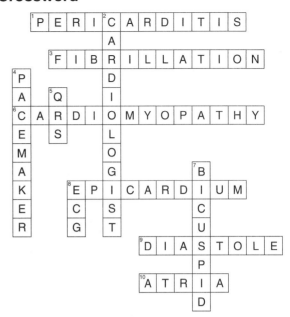

Check Your Knowledge
Multiple Choice
1. C, p. 380
2. D, p. 384
3. C, p. 386
4. D, p. 376
5. C, p. 376
6. B, p. 376
7. D, p. 378
8. A, p. 382
9. C, p. 386
10. D, p. 388

Matching
11. F, p. 381
12. G, p. 384
13. H, p. 379
14. I, p. 380
15. J, p. 378
16. B, p. 376
17. C, p. 376
18. A, p. 386
19. D, p. 384
20. E, p. 381

The Heart

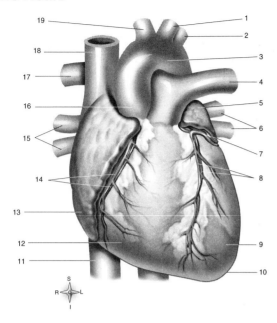

Conduction System of the Heart

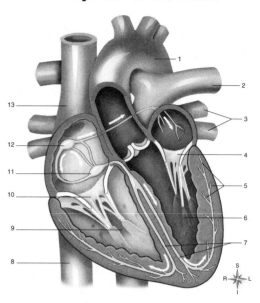

1. Left common carotid artery
2. Left subclavian artery
3. Arch of aorta
4. Left pulmonary artery
5. Left atrium
6. Left pulmonary veins
7. Great cardiac vein
8. Branches of left coronary artery and cardiac vein
9. Left ventricle
10. Apex
11. Inferior vena cava
12. Right ventricle
13. Right atrium
14. Right coronary artery and cardiac vein
15. Right pulmonary veins
16. Ascending aorta
17. Right pulmonary artery
18. Superior vena cava
19. Brachiocephalic trunk

1. Aorta
2. Pulmonary artery
3. Pulmonary veins
4. Mitral (bicuspid) valve
5. Purkinje fibers
6. Left ventricle
7. Right and left branches of AV bundle block (bundle of His)
8. Inferior vena cava
9. Right ventricle
10. Tricuspid valve
11. Atrioventricular (AV) node
12. Superior (SA) node (pacemaker)
13. Superior vena cava

Normal ECG Deflections

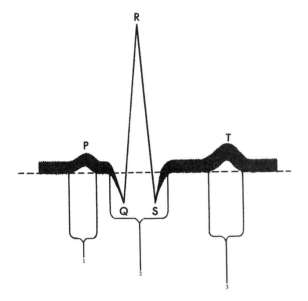

1. Atrial depolarization
2. Ventricular depolarization
3. Ventricular repolarization

CHAPTER 14
The Circulation of the Blood

Matching
1. D, p. 396
2. B, p. 396
3. C, p. 396
4. G, p. 396
5. A, p. 396
6. E, p. 396
7. F, p. 396

Matching
8. I, p. 400
9. B, p. 400
10. D, p 400
11. E, p. 400
12. A, p. 400
13. C, p. 401
14. F, p. 402
15. G, p. 402
16. J, p. 402
17. H, p. 401

Circle the Correct Answer
18. D, p. 402
19. C, p. 403
20. B, p. 403
21. B, p. 403
22. D, p. 404

23. B, p. 406
24. B, p. 406
25. A, p. 406
26. D, p. 403

True or False
27. F (Highest/arteries; lowest/veins), p. 406
28. F (Blood pressure gradient), p. 406
29. F (Stop), p. 406
30. F (High blood pressure), p. 408
31. F (Decreases), p. 408
32. T
33. T
34. T
35. F (Increases blood pressure/weaker heartbeat tends to decrease it), p. 408
36. F (Contract), p. 410
37. F (decreases), p. 409
38. T
39. T
40. F (Right), p. 410
41. F (Artery), p. 411
42. T
43. T
44. F (Brachial), p 412

Fill in the Blanks
45. Septic shock, p. 414
46. Cardiogenic shock, p. 413
47. Anaphylaxis; anaphylactic shock, p. 413
48. Neurogenic shock, p. 413
49. Low blood volume, p. 413
50. Toxic shock syndrome, p. 414

Unscramble the Words
51. Systemic
52. Venule
53. Artery
54. Pulse
55. Vessel

Applying What You Know
56. Anaphylactic shock
57. Hypovolemic shock
58. Varicose veins; wear support stockings
59. Hemorrhage

60. **WORD FIND**

Y	H	Y	S	I	S	O	B	M	O	R	H	T	A	R
L	A	C	I	L	I	B	M	U	O	A	Y	N	I	Y
E	E	S	Y	S	T	E	M	I	C	C	G	D	E	U
M	V	E	N	U	L	E	D	D	C	I	X	M	D	I
E	Y	M	U	I	R	T	A	R	N	L	E	C	G	Y
N	O	I	T	A	Z	I	R	A	L	O	P	E	D	N
U	D	L	A	T	R	O	P	C	I	T	A	P	E	H
S	I	U	K	M	U	E	T	O	E	S	L	U	P	U
R	P	N	F	Y	C	B	E	D	R	A	L	Z	P	J
D	S	A	H	T	I	T	V	N	L	I	I	B	D	W
Q	U	R	O	I	V	A	Q	E	O	D	A	K	R	K
K	C	R	M	P	G	A	I	G	N	D	D	Z	Y	J
Y	I	Y	R	I	N	E	A	F	Z	L	Q	S	P	X
S	R	M	I	C	C	Q	O	A	W	U	N	H	O	K
P	T	A	V	H	H	Z	L	H	I	J	J	X	K	Z

Crossword

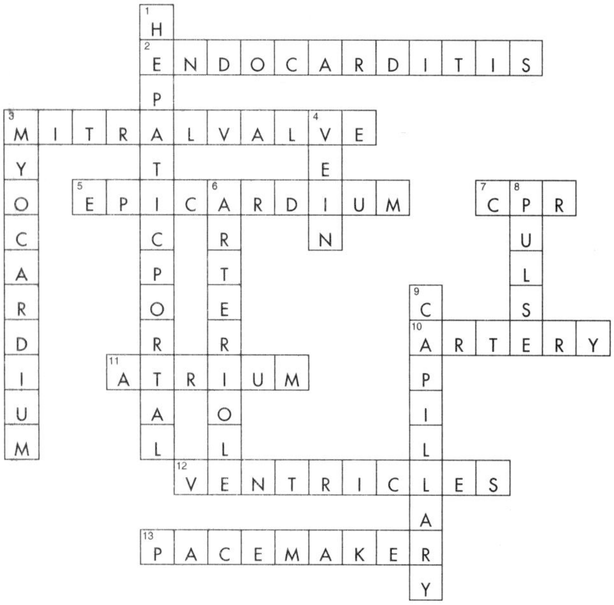

Check Your Knowledge
Multiple Choice

1. C, p. 412
2. A, p. 414
3. C, p. 413
4. C, p. 396
5. C, p. 396
6. B, p. 402
7. A, p. 406
8. A, p. 408
9. D, p. 400
10. B, p. 400

Matching

11. G, p. 396
12. A, p. 400
13. I, p. 402
14. C, p. 406
15. F, p. 401
16. B, p. 402
17. H, p. 403
18. D, p. 401
19. E, p. 396
20. J, p. 413

Fetal Circulation

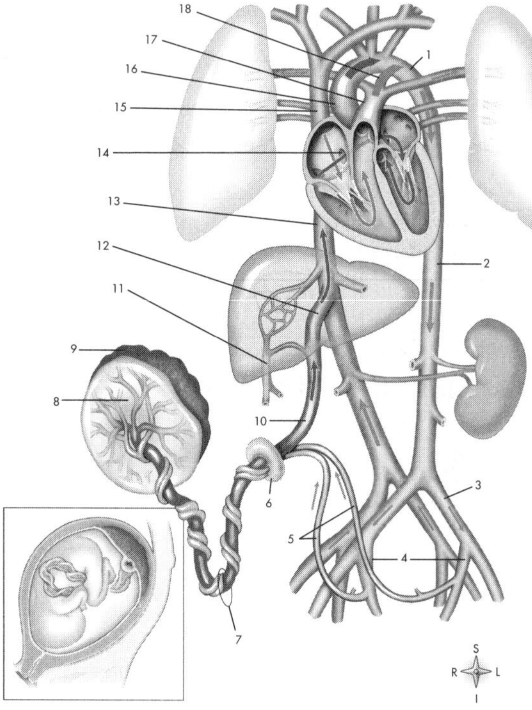

1. Aortic arch
2. Abdominal aorta
3. Common iliac artery
4. Internal iliac arteries
5. Umbilical arteries
6. Fetal umbilicus
7. Umbilical cord
8. Fetal side of placenta
9. Maternal side of placenta
10. Umbilical vein
11. Hepatic portal vein
12. Ductus venosus
13. Inferior vena cava
14. Foramen ovale
15. Superior vena cava
16. Ascending aorta
17. Pulmonary trunk
18. Ductus arteriosus

Hepatic Portal Circulation

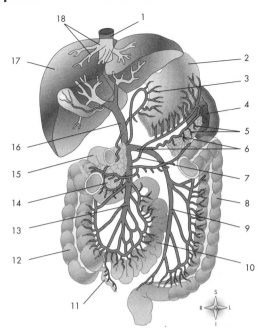

1. Inferior vena cava
2. Stomach
3. Gastric vein
4. Spleen
5. Pancreatic vein
6. Splenic vein
7. Gastroepiploic vein
8. Descending colon
9. Inferior mesenteric vein
10. Small intestine
11. Appendix
12. Ascending colon
13. Superior mesenteric vein
14. Pancreas
15. Duodenum
16. Hepatic portal vein
17. Liver
18. Hepatic veins

Principal Arteries of the Body

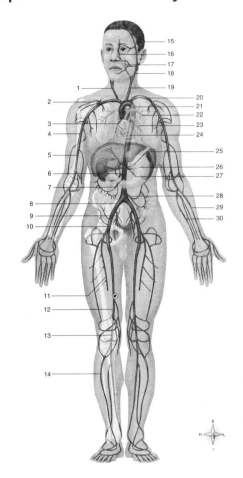

1. Right common carotid
2. Brachiocephalic
3. Right coronary
4. Axillary
5. Brachial
6. Superior mesenteric
7. Abdominal aorta
8. Common iliac
9. Internal iliac
10. External iliac
11. Deep femoral
12. Femoral
13. Popliteal
14. Anterior tibial
15. Occipital
16. Facial
17. Internal carotid
18. External carotid
19. Left common carotid
20. Left subclavian
21. Arch of aorta
22. Pulmonary
23. Left coronary
24. Aorta
25. Splenic
26. Renal
27. Celiac
28. Inferior mesenteric
29. Radial
30. Ulnar

Principal Veins of the Body

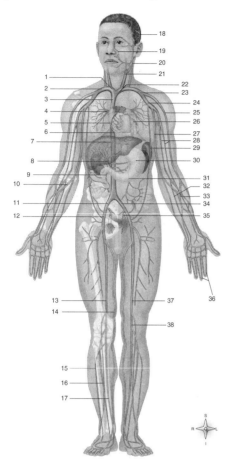

1. Right brachiocephalic
2. Right subclavian
3. Superior vena cava
4. Right pulmonary
5. Small cardiac
6. Inferior vena cava
7. Hepatic
8. Hepatic portal
9. Superior mesenteric
10. Median cubital
11. Common iliac
12. External iliac
13. Femoral
14. Great saphenous
15. Fibular (peroneal)
16. Anterior tibial
17. Posterior tibial
18. Occipital
19. Facial
20. External jugular
21. Internal jugular
22. Left brachiocephalic
23. Left subclavian
24. Axillary
25. Cephalic
26. Great cardiac
27. Basilic
28. Brachial veins
29. Long thoracic
30. Splenic
31. Inferior mesenteric
32. Ulnar vein
33. Radial vein
34. Common iliac
35. Internal iliac
36. Digital veins

CHAPTER 15
The Lymphatic System and Immunity

Fill in the Blanks
1. Lymph, p. 422
2. Interstitial fluid, p. 422
3. Lymphatic capillaries, p. 422
4. Right lymphatic duct and thoracic duct, p. 423
5. Cisterna chyli, p. 423
6. Lymph nodes, p. 424
7. Afferent, p. 426
8. Efferent, p. 426
9. Lymphedema, p. 424
10. Lymphoma, p. 427

Choose the Correct Response
11. B, p. 428
12. C, p. 428
13. C, p. 428
14. A, p. 427
15. C, p. 428
16. A, p. 427
17. A, p. 427

Matching
18. C, p. 429
19. A, p. 430
20. E, p. 430
21. B, p. 430
22. D, p. 430

Matching
23. C, p. 431
24. A, p. 432
25. F, p. 432
26. B, p. 432
27. G, p. 432
28. D, p. 433
29. H, p. 431
30. E, p. 433

Multiple Choice
31. D, p. 434
32. D, p. 435
33. C, p. 435
34. C, p. 435
35. C, p. 435
36. E, p. 435
37. E, p. 435
38. C, p. 435
39. E, p. 435
40. E, p. 436
41. A, p. 435
42. B, p. 436

Circle the Correct Answer

43. Hypersensitivity, p. 438
44. Allergens, p. 438
45. Anaphylactic shock, p. 438
46. Lupus, p. 439
47. Isoimmunity, p. 439
48. HLAs, p. 439

Select the Correct Response

49. B, p. 441
50. A, p. 441
51. A, p. 441
52. B, p. 441
53. A, p. 441

Unscramble the Words

54. Complement
55. Immunity
56. Clones
57. Interferon
58. Memory cells

Applying What You Know

59. Natural active immunity
60. AIDS
61. Baby Wilson had no means of producing T cells, thus making him susceptible to several diseases. Isolation was a means of controlling his exposure to these diseases.

62. **WORD FIND**

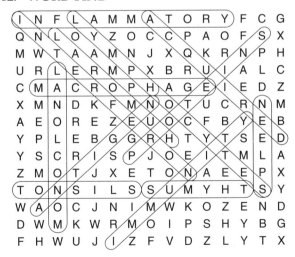

Crossword

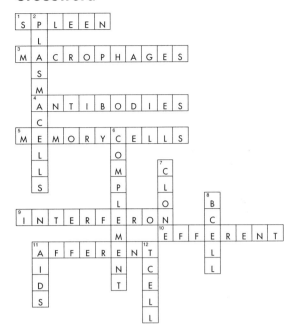

Check Your Knowledge
Multiple Choice

1. A, p. 436
2. A, p. 422
3. D, p. 441
4. B, p. 440
5. D, p. 435
6. B, p. 433
7. D, p. 433
8. D, p. 434
9. D, p. 431
10. C, p. 430

Matching

11. E, p. 428
12. D, p. 435
13. I, p. 435
14. H, p. 441
15. G, p. 433
16. B, p. 424
17. A, p. 423
18. J, p. 436
19. C, p. 430
20. F, p. 432

Principal Organs of the Lymphatic System

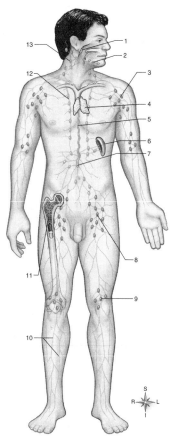

1. Tonsils
2. Submandibular nodes
3. Axillary lymph nodes
4. Thymus
5. Thoracic duct
6. Spleen
7. Cisterna chyli
8. Inguinal lymph nodes
9. Popliteal lymph nodes
10. Lymph vessels
11. Red bone marrow
12. Right lymphatic duct
13. Cervical lymph nodes

CHAPTER 16
The Respiratory System

Matching
1. J, p. 453
2. G, p. 456
3. A, p. 455
4. I, p. 456
5. B, p. 456
6. F, p. 456
7. C, p. 456
8. H, p. 456
9. D, p. 456
10. E, p. 453

Fill in the Blanks
11. Air distributor, p. 453
12. Gas exchanger, p. 453
13. Filters, p. 454
14. Warms, p. 454
15. Humidifies, p. 454
16. Nose, p. 454
17. Pharynx, p. 454
18. Larynx, p. 454
19. Trachea, p. 454
20. Bronchi, p. 454
21. Lungs, p. 454
22. Alveoli, p. 454
23. Diffusion, p. 455
24. Respiratory membrane, p. 455
25. Surface, p. 455

Circle the One That Does Not Belong
26. Oropharynx (the others refer to the nose)
27. Conchae (the others refer to paranasal sinuses)
28. Epiglottis (the others refer to the pharynx)
29. Uvula (the others refer to the adenoids)
30. Larynx (the others refer to the eustachian tubes)
31. Tonsils (the others refer to the larynx)
32. Eustachian tube (the others refer to the tonsils)
33. Pharynx (the others refer to the larynx)

Choose the Correct Response
34. A, p. 457
35. B, p. 458
36. A, p. 457
37. A, p. 457
38. A, p. 457
39. B, p. 458
40. B, p. 458
41. C, p. 460
42. A, p. 461
43. B, p. 461
44. A, p. 461

Fill in the Blanks
45. Trachea, p. 463
46. C-rings of cartilage, p. 463
47. Heimlich maneuver, p. 462
48. Primary bronchi, p. 463
49. Alveolar sacs, p. 464
50. Apex, p. 465
51. Pleura, p. 465
52. Pleurisy, p. 466
53. Pneumothorax, p. 466

True or False

54. F (Breathing), p. 467
55. F (Expiration), p. 468
56. F (Down), p. 468
57. F (Internal respiration), p. 470
58. T
59. F (1 pint), p. 471.
60. T
61. F (Vital capacity), p. 472
62. T

Multiple Choice

63. E, p. 467
64. C, p. 470
65. C, p. 468
66. B, p. 467
67. D, p. 472
68. D, p. 472
69. D, p. 472

Matching

70. E, p. 473
71. B, p. 474
72. G, p. 474
73. A, p. 474
74. F, p. 474
75. D, p. 474
76. C, p. 474

Fill in the Blanks

77. Pneumonia, p. 475
78. Tuberculosis, p. 475
79. Emphysema, p. 478
80. Asthma, p. 478

Unscramble the Words

81. Pleurisy
82. Bronchitis
83. Epistaxis
84. Adenoids
85. Inspiration

Applying What You Know

86. During the day, Mr. Gorski's cilia are paralyzed because of his heavy smoking. They use the time when Mr. Gorski is asleep to sweep accumulations of mucus and bacteria toward the pharynx. When Mr. Gorski awakens, these collections are waiting to be eliminated.
87. Impossible for air to travel from the nose into the throat. The individual may be forced to breathe through the mouth.
88. During expiration, the alveoli are unable to force out a normal amount of air. Residual volume is increased at the expense of the expi-

ratory reserve volume. Pulmonary infections can cause inflammation and an accumulation of fluid in the air spaces of the lungs. The fluid reduces the amount of space available for air and thus decreases the vital capacity.

89. **WORD FIND**

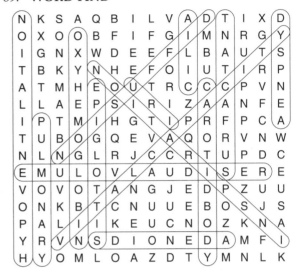

Crossword

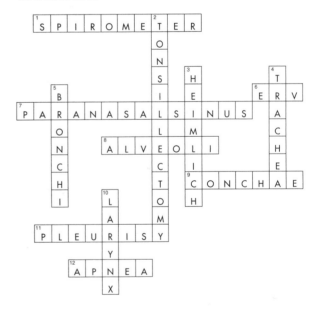

Check Your Knowledge
Multiple Choice

1. A, p. 474
2. B, p. 458
3. D, p. 465
4. B, p. 472
5. A, p. 465
6. D, p. 460
7. A, p. 463
8. C, p. 468

9. D, p. 467
10. B, p. 467

Matching

11. E, p. 460
12. I, p. 467
13. A, p. 465
14. G, p. 466
15. D, p. 477
16. B, p. 458
17. C, p. 457
18. H, p. 463
19. F, p. 468
20. J, p. 464

Sagittal View of Face and Neck

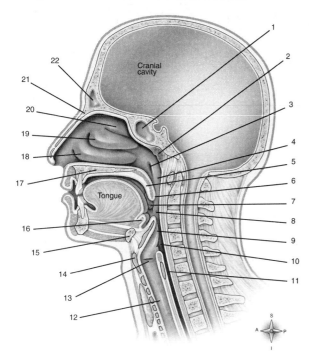

1. Sphenoidal sinus
2. Pharyngeal tonsil (adenoids)
3. Opening of auditory (eustachian) tube
4. Nasopharynx
5. Soft palate
6. Uvula
7. Palatine tonsil
8. Oropharynx
9. Epiglottis (part of larynx)
10. Laryngopharynx
11. Esophagus
12. Trachea
13. Vocal cords (part of larynx)
14. Thyroid cartilage (part of larynx)
15. Hyoid bone
16. Lingual tonsil
17. Hard palate
18. Inferior concha
19. Middle nasal concha of ethmoid
20. Superior nasal concha of ethmoid
21. Nasal bone
22. Frontal sinus

Respiratory Organs

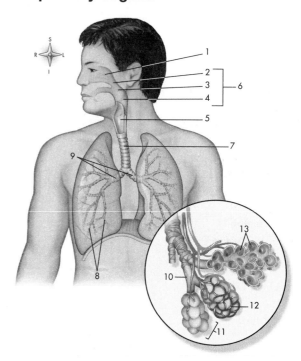

1. Nasal cavity
2. Nasopharynx
3. Oropharynx
4. Laryngopharynx
5. Pharynx
6. Larynx
7. Trachea
8. Bronchioles
9. Left and right primary bronchi
10. Alveolar duct
11. Alveolar sac
12. Capillary
13. Alveoli

Pulmonary Ventilation Volumes

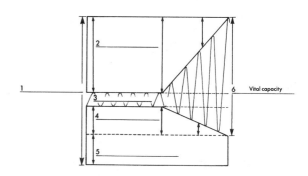

1. Total lung capacity
2. Inspiratory reserve volume
3. Tidal volume
4. Expiratory reserve volume
5. Residual volume
6. Vital capacity

CHAPTER 17
The Digestive System

Fill in the Blanks
1. Gastrointestinal tract or GI tract, p. 487
2. Mechanical, p. 487
3. Chemical, p. 487
4. Feces, p. 488
5. Digestion, absorption, and metabolism, p. 488

Select the Correct Response
6. A, p. 488
7. B, p. 488
8. B, p. 488
9. A, p. 488
10. A, p. 488
11. A, p. 488
12. A, p. 488
13. A, p. 488
14. B, p. 488
15. B, p. 488
16. B, p. 488
17. B, p. 488

Multiple Choice
18. E, p. 489
19. C, p. 490
20. E, p. 490
21. D, p. 491
22. B, p. 490
23. C, p. 490
24. D, p. 490
25. D, p. 490
26. D, p. 492
27. A, p. 494
28. C, p. 494
29. A, p. 494
30. A, P. 490
31. B, p. 490
32. C, p. 490

Fill in the Blanks
33. Visceral peritoneum, p. 496
34. Mouth; anus, p. 495
35. Lumen, p. 496
36. Mucosa, p. 496
37. Submucosa, p. 496
38. Peristalsis, p. 496
39. Serosa, p. 496
40. Mesentery, p. 496

Fill in the Blanks
41. Pharynx, p. 495
42. Esophagus, p. 496
43. Stomach, p. 496

44. Lower esophageal sphincter, p. 497
45. Chyme, p. 498
46. Fundus, p. 498
47. Body, p. 498
48. Pylorus, p. 498
49. Pyloric sphincter, p. 499
50. Small intestine, p. 499

Matching
51. D, p. 498
52. J, p. 499
53. G, p. 497
54. A, p. 496
55. H, p. 501
56. B, p. 498
57. C, p. 496
58. E, p. 500
59. I, p. 497
60. F, p. 499

Multiple Choice
61. C, p. 501
62. B, p. 501
63. A, p. 504
64. A, p. 505
65. B, p. 504
66. E, p. 503
67. D, p. 505
68. D, p. 504
69. B, p. 504
70. C, p. 504

True or False
71. F (Vitamin K), p. 508
72. F (No villi are present in the large intestine), p. 508
73. F (Diarrhea), p. 510
74. F (Cecum), p. 509
75. F (Hepatic), p. 509
76. F (Sigmoid), p. 509
77. T
78. T
79. F (Parietal), p. 512
80. F (Mesentery), p. 513
81. F (Diverticulitis), p. 510
82. T
83. T
84. F (Ascites), p. 513

Multiple Choice
85. B, p. 515
86. D, p. 515
87. C, p. 515
88. C, p. 514
89. C, p. 514

Chemical Digestion

90.   Fill in the blank areas on the chart below.

DIGESTIVE JUICES AND ENZYMES	SUBSTANCE DIGESTED (OR HYDROLYZED)	RESULTING PRODUCT
Saliva		
1.	1. Starch (polysaccharide)	1.
Gastric Juice		
2.	2.	2. Partially digested proteins
Pancreatic Juice		
3.	3.	3. Peptides and amino acids
4.	4. Fats emulsified by bile	4.
5.	5. Starch	5.
Intestinal Enzymes		
6.	6. Peptides	6.
7. Sucrase	7.	7.
8.	8. Lactose	8.
9.	9.	9. Glucose

Unscramble the Words

91.   Bolus
92.   Chyme
93.   Papilla
94.   Peritoneum
95.   Lace apron

Applying What You Know

96.   Ulcer
97.   Pylorospasm
98.   Cholelithiasis; cholecystectomy

99.   **WORD FIND**

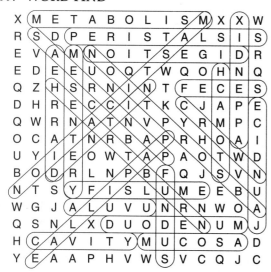

Crossword

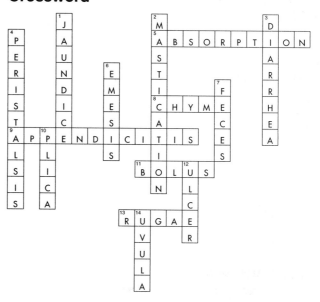

Check Your Knowledge
Multiple Choice

1.   A, p. 505
2.   C, p. 498
3,   A, p. 501
4.   B, p. 491
5.   B, p. 496
6.   B, p. 500
7.   B, p. 513
8.   C, p. 514

9. C, p. 514
10. A, p. 515

Completion

11. N, p. 508
12. J, p. 513
13. P, p. 514
14. Q, R, A, p. 501
15. W, p. 504
16. H, K, D, p. 488
17. E, p. 504
18. T, U, C, X, p. 496
19. G, p. 497
20. I, O, S, F, p. 490

Tooth

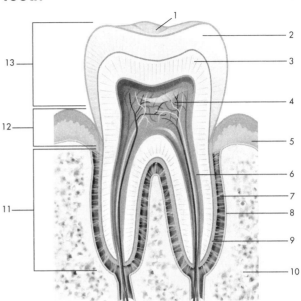

1. Cusp
2. Enamel
3. Dentin
4. Pulp cavity with nerves and vessels
5. Gingiva (gum)
6. Root canal
7. Periodontal ligament
8. Periodontal membrane
9. Cementum
10. Bone
11. Root
12. Neck
13. Crown

Location of Digestive Organs

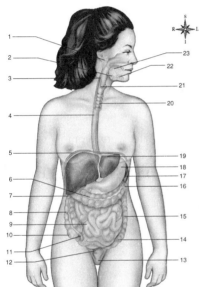

1. Parotid gland
2. Submandibular salivary gland
3. Pharynx
4. Esophagus
5. Diaphragm
6. Transverse colon
7. Hepatic flexure of colon
8. Ascending colon
9. Ileum
10. Cecum
11. Vermiform appendix
12. Rectum
13. Anal canal
14. Sigmoid colon
15. Descending colon
16. Splenic flexure of colon
17. Spleen
18. Stomach

19. Liver
20. Trachea
21. Larynx
22. Sublingual salivary gland
23. Tongue
24. Common hepatic duct

25. Cystic duct
26. Gallbladder
27. Duodenum
28. Pancreas
29. Stomach
30. Spleen
31. Liver

The Salivary Glands

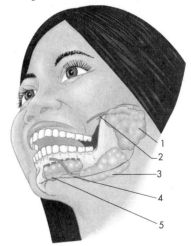

1. Parotid gland
2. Parotid duct
3. Submandibular gland
4. Submandibular duct
5. Sublingual gland

Stomach

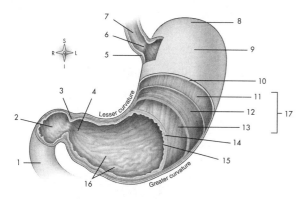

1. Duodenum
2. Duodenal bulb
3. Pyloric sphincter
4. Pylorus
5. Lower esophageal sphincter
6. Gastroesophageal sphincter
7. Esophagus
8. Fundus
9. Body of stomach
10. Serosa
11. Longitudinal muscle layer
12. Circular muscle layer
13. Oblique muscle layer
14. Submucosa
15. Mucosa
16. Rugae
17. Muscularis

Gallbladder and Bile Ducts

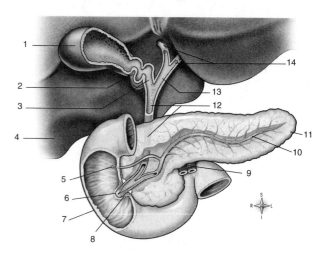

1. Corpus (body) of gallbladder
2. Neck of gallbladder
3. Cystic duct
4. Liver
5. Minor duodenal papilla
6. Major duodenal papilla
7. Duodenum
8. Sphincter muscles
9. Superior mesenteric artery and vein
10. Pancreatic duct
11. Pancreas
12. Common bile duct
13. Common hepatic duct
14. Right and left hepatic ducts

The Small Intestine

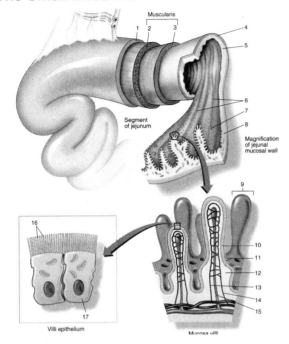

The Large Intestine

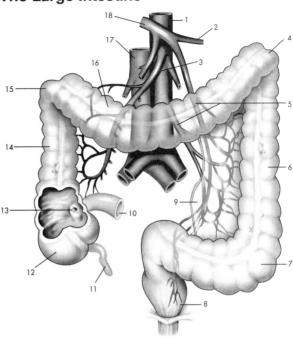

1. Serosa
2. Longitudinal muscle (Answer #2 and answer #3 constitute the "muscularis")
3. Circular muscle (Answer #2 and answer #3 constitute the "muscularis")
4. Submucosa
5. Mucosa
6. Plica (fold)
7. Lymph node
8. Mucosa
9. Single villus
10. Epithelium
11. Microvilli
12. Mucosa
13. Vein
14. Artery
15. Lacteal (lymph)
16. Microvilli
17. Epithelial cell

1. Aorta
2. Splenic vein
3. Superior mesenteric artery
4. Splenic (left colic) flexure
5. Inferior mesenteric artery and vein
6. Descending colon
7. Sigmoid colon
8. Rectum
9. Mesentery
10. Ileum
11. Vermiform appendix
12. Cecum
13. Ileocecal valve
14. Ascending colon
15. Hepatic (right colic) flexure
16. Transverse colon
17. Inferior vena cava
18. Portal vein

CHAPTER 18
Nutrition and Metabolism

Fill in the Blanks
1. Bile, p. 526
2. Prothrombin, p. 526
3. Fibrinogen, p. 526
4. Iron, p. 526
5. Hepatic portal vein, p. 526

Matching
6. B, p. 528
7. A, p. 526

8. C, p. 529
9. D, p. 530
10. E, p. 531
11. A, p. 527
12. E, p. 531
13. A, p. 527

Circle the Word that Does Not Belong

14. Bile (all others refer to carbohydrate metabolism)
15. Amino acids (all others refer to fat metabolism)
16. M (all others refer to vitamins)
17. Iron (all others refer to protein metabolism)
18. Insulin (all others tend to increase blood glucose)
19. Folic acid (all others are minerals)
20. Ascorbic acid (all others refer to the B-complex vitamins)

Multiple Choice

21. C, p. 532
22. A, p. 532
23. A, p. 534
24. D, p. 532
25. D, p. 532

Choose the Correct Response

26. B, p. 532
27. C, p. 533
28. G, p. 534
29. F, p. 533
30. A, p. 532
31. H, p. 534
32. E, p. 533
33. D, p. 533

Multiple Choice

34. C, p. 534
35. B, p. 534
36. B, p. 535
37. A, p. 535
38. C, p. 535
39. D, p. 535

True or False

40. T
41. F (Hypothermia), p. 536
42. T
43. F (Heat stroke), p. 536
44. F (Malignant hyperthermia), p. 536

Unscramble the Words

45. Liver
46. Catabolism
47. Amino
48. Pyruvic
49. Evaporation

Applying What You Know

50. Weight loss and anorexia nervosa
51. Iron; meat, eggs, vegetables, and legumes
52. He was carbohydrate loading or glycogen loading, which allows the muscles to sustain aerobic exercise for up to 50% longer than usual.

53. **WORD FIND**

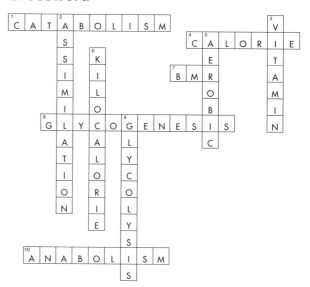

Crossword

Check Your Knowledge
Multiple Choice

1. B, p. 527
2. A, p. 528
3. C, p. 528
4. C, p. 532
5. B, p. 532

6. B, p. 528
7. A, p. 528
8. A, p. 534
9. B, p. 526
10. D, p. 526

Completion

11. C, D, I, p. 525
12. E, p. 527
13. J, p. 527
14. G, p. 527
15. B, p. 528
16. D, p. 528
17. L, p. 528
18. A, p. 530
19. K, H, p. 531
20. F, p. 525

CHAPTER 19
The Urinary System

Multiple Choice

1. E, p. 544
2. C, p. 547
3. E, p. 547
4. C, p. 548
5. E, p. 550
6. C, p. 550
7. B, p. 550
8. E, p. 550
9. C, p. 550
10. C, p. 551
11. B, p. 551 (Review Chapter 11)
12. D, p. 551

Choose the Correct Term

13. G, p. 545
14. I, p. 548
15. H, p. 548
16. B, p. 544
17. K, p. 547
18. F, p. 545
19. J, p. 547
20. D, p. 545
21. L, p. 547
22. C, p. 545
23. E, p. 545
24. A, p. 545

Choose the Correct Term

25. C, p. 554
26. B, p. 554
27. C, p. 554
28. A, p. 553

29. B, p. 554
30. C, p. 554
31. C, p. 554
32. A, p. 553
33. C, p. 554 Figure 19-8
34. B, p. 554
35. A, p. 553
36. B, p. 554

Fill in the Blanks

37. Urinalysis, p. 553
38. Mucous membrane, p. 554
39. Centrifuge, p. 553
40. Anuria, p. 552
41. Cystitis or bladder infections, p. 555
42. Semen, p. 554
43. Urinary meatus, p. 554

Fill in the Blanks

44. Micturition, p. 554
45. Urination, p. 554
46. Voiding, p. 554
47. Internal urethral sphincter, p. 555
48. Exit, p. 555
49. Urethra, p. 555
50. Voluntary, p. 555
51. Emptying reflex, p. 555
52. Urethra, p. 555
53. Retention, p. 556
54. Suppression, p. 556
55. Stress incontinence, p. 556

Select the Correct Answer

56. I, p. 556
57. C, p. 557
58. G, p. 556
59. F, p. 557
60. K, p. 558
61. A, p. 558
62. H, p. 559
63. J, p. 559
64. B, p. 557
65. D, p. 559
66. E, p. 558
67. L, p. 558

Unscramble the Words

68. Calyx
69. Voiding
70. Papilla
71. Glomerulus
72. Pyramids

Applying What You Know

73. Polyuria

74. Residual urine is often the cause of repeated cystitis.
75. A high percentage of catheterized patients develop cystitis, often due to poor aseptic technique when inserting the catheter.
76. Hemorrhage causes a drop in blood pressure, which decreases the urine output and can eventually lead to kidney failure.

77. **WORD FIND**

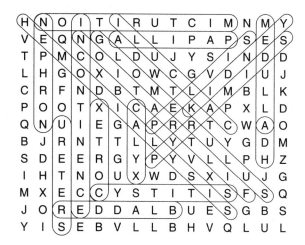

Crossword

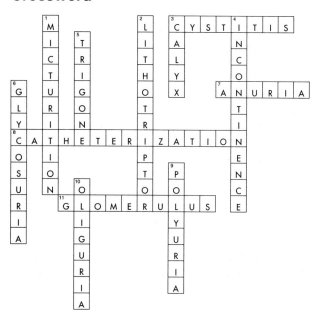

Check Your Knowledge
Multiple Choice

1. D, p. 555
2. B, p. 561
3. D, p. 543
4. A, p. 551
5. C, p. 556
6. C, p. 550

7. B, p. 555
8. C, p. 553
9. B, p. 547
10. A, p. 545

Matching

11. E, p. 556
12. C, p. 552
13. F, p. 558
14. D, p. 554
15. J, p. 552
16. H, p. 552
17. A, p. 556
18. G, p. 557
19. I, p. 556
20. B, p. 550

Urinary System

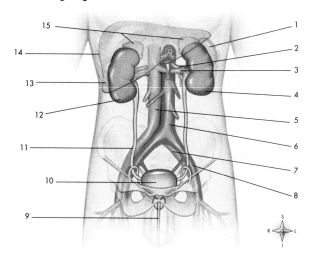

1. Spleen
2. Renal artery
3. Renal vein
4. Left kidney
5. Inferior vena cava
6. Abdominal aorta
7. Common iliac vein
8. Common iliac artery
9. Urethra
10. Urinary bladder
11. Ureter
12. Right kidney
13. Twelfth rib
14. Liver
15. Adrenal glands

Kidney

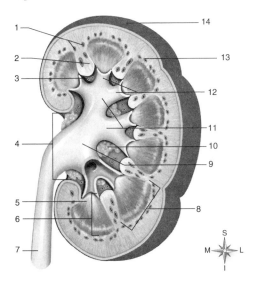

1. Interlobular arteries
2. Renal column
3. Renal sinus
4. Hilum
5. Renal papilla of pyramid
6. Medulla
7. Ureter
8. Medullary pyramid
9. Renal pelvis
10. Fat
11. Major calyces
12. Minor calyces
13. Cortex
14. Capsule (fibrous)

Nephron

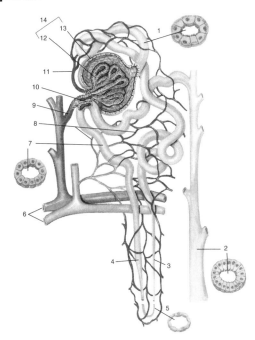

1. Proximal convoluted tubule
2. Collecting duct
3. Descending limb of Henle loop
4. Ascending limb of Henle loop
5. Descending limb of Henle loop
6. Artery and vein
7. Distal convoluted tubule
8. Peritubular capillaries
9. Afferent arteriole
10. Juxtaglomerular (JG) apparatus
11. Efferent arteriole
12. Glomerulus
13. Bowman capsule
14. Renal corpuscle

CHAPTER 20
Fluid and Electrolyte Balance

Circle the Correct Answer
1. Inside, p. 571
2. Extracellular, p. 571
3. Extracellular, p. 571
4. Lower, p. 570
5. More, p. 571
6. Decline, p. 571
7. Less, p. 571
8. Decreases, p. 571
9. 55%, p. 570
10. Fluid balance, p. 569

Multiple Choice

11. A, p. 574
12. D, p. 574
13. A, p. 574
14. C, p. 573
15. E, p. 573
16. D, p. 573
17. D, p. 572
18. C, p. 576
19. B, p. 572
20. D, p. 578
21. E, p. 576
22. B, p. 577
23. B, p. 577
24. B, p. 577

True or False

25. F (Catabolism), p. 572
26. T
27. T
28. F (Nonelectrolyte), p. 574
29. T
30. F (Hypervolemia), p. 575 , Figure 20-7
31. F (Tubular function), p. 578
32. F (2400 ml), p. 573
33. T
34. F (100 mEq), p. 576

Fill in the Blanks

35. Dehydration, p. 577
36. Decreases, p. 577
37. Decrease, p. 577
38. Overhydration, p. 578
39. Intravenous fluids, p. 578
40. Heart, p. 578
41. Hypernatremia, p. 579
42. Hyperkalemia, p. 579

Unscramble the Words

43. Edema
44. Fluid
45. Ion
46. Intravenous
47. Volume

Applying What You Know

48. Ms. Titus could not accurately measure water intake created by foods or catabolism, nor could she measure output created by lungs, skin, or the intestines.
49. A careful record of fluid intake and output should be maintained, and the patient should be monitored for signs and symptoms of electrolyte and water imbalance.
50. Jack's body contained more water. Obese people have a lower water content than slender people.

51. **WORD FIND**

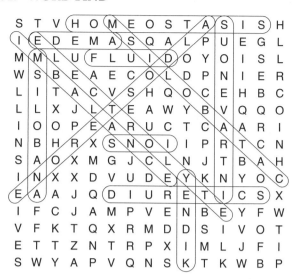

Crossword

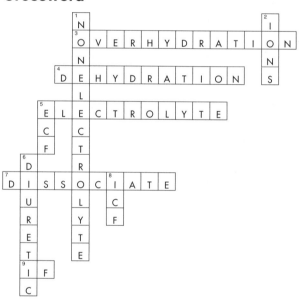

Check Your Knowledge
Multiple Choice

1. A, p. 570
2. D, p. 572
3. D, p. 577
4. C, p. 577
5. A, p. 576
6. B, p. 575
7. D, p. 573
8. A, p. 576
9. A, p. 574
10. D, p. 575

Completion

11. E, p. 578

12. B, p. 575
13. J, M, K, p. 571
14. F, p. 574
15. D, p. 572
16. L, p. 572
17. I, p. 577
18. C, p. 577
19. H and A, p. 572
20. N, p. 569

CHAPTER 21
Acid-Base Balance

Choose the Correct Term
1. B, p. 588
2. A, p. 588
3. A, p. 588
4 B, p. 588
5. B, p. 588
6. B, p. 588
7. B, p. 588
8. A, p. 588
9. B, p. 588
10. B, p. 588

Multiple Choice
11. E, p. 589
12. E, p. 589
13. A, p. 589
14. E, p. 590
15. C, p. 590
16. D, p. 590
17. C, p. 592
18. B, p. 592
19. D, p. 592
20. E, p. 594
21. E, p. 594

True or False
22. F (Buffer instead of heart), p. 588
23. F (Buffer pairs), p. 589
24. T
25. T
26. F (Alkalosis), p. 592
27. F (Reverse—arterial blood has a higher pH), p. 588
28. T
29. F (Kidneys), p. 594
30. F (Lungs), p. 594

Matching
31. E, p. 595
32. G, p. 596
33. F, p. 595

34. A, p. 594
35. I, p. 595
36. B, p. 596
37. H, p. 596
38. C, p. 596
39. D, p. 596
40. J, p. 596

Applying What You Know
41. Normal saline contains chloride ions, which replace bicarbonate ions and thus relieve the bicarbonate excess that occurs during severe vomiting.
42. Most citrus fruits, although acid-tasting, are fully oxidized with the help of buffers during metabolism and have little effect on acid-base balance. Cranberry juice is one of the few exceptions.
43. Milk of magnesia. It is a base. Interestingly, milk is slightly acidic.

44. **WORD FIND**

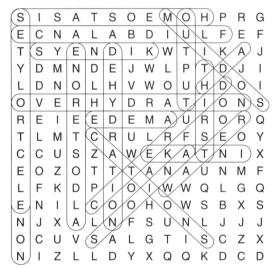

Crossword

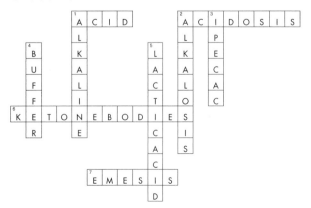

Check Your Knowledge
Multiple Choice

1. A, p. 589
2. C, p. 594
3. A, p. 592
4. D, p. 588
5. A, p. 596
6. D, p. 596
7. D, p. 590
8. D, p. 595
9. D, p. 589
10. A, p. 590

Matching

11. G, p. 588
12. C, p. 588
13. I, p. 589
14. E, p. 596
15. F, p. 596
16. A, p. 594
17. B, p. 596
18. D, p. 590
19. J, p. 589
20. H, p. 596

CHAPTER 22
The Reproductive Systems

Matching
Group A

1. D, p. 605
2. C, p. 604
3. E, p. 604
4. B, p. 605
5. A, p. 604

Group B

6. C, p. 605
7. A, p. 605
8. D, p. 604
9. B, p. 605
10. E, p. 605

Multiple Choice

11. B, p. 605
12. C, p. 605
13. A, p. 605
14. D, p. 605
15. E, p. 605
16. D, p. 608
17. C, p. 609
18. C, p. 605
19. A, p. 608

Fill in the Blanks

20. Testes, p. 604
21. Spermatozoa or sperm, p. 605
22. Ovum, p. 604
23. Testosterone, p. 605
24. Interstitial cells, p. 605
25. Masculinizing, p. 609
26. Anabolic, p. 609

Choose the Correct Term

27. B, p. 609
28. H, p. 610
29. G, p. 610
30. A, p. 609
31. F, p. 610
32. C, p. 610
33. I, p. 610
34. E, p. 610
35. D, p. 611
36. J, p. 611

Fill in the Blanks

37. Oligospermia, p. 612
38. 2 months, p. 612
39. Cryptorchidism, p. 612
40. Benign prostatic hypertrophy, p. 612
41. Phimosis, p. 611
42. Impotence or erectile dysfunction, p. 613
43. Hydrocele, p. 613
44. Inguinal hernia, p. 614
45. Prostate, p. 613

Matching

46. D, p. 614
47. C, p. 614
48. B, p. 614
49. A, p. 614
50. E, p. 614

Choose the Correct Structure

51. A, p. 619
52. B, p. 618
53. A, p. 619
54. B, p. 617
55. A, p. 619
56. A, p. 619
57. A, p. 619
58. B, p. 614

Fill in the Blanks

59. Gonads, p. 614
60. Oogenesis, p. 616
61. Meiosis, p. 616
62. One-half (or 23), p. 616
63. Fertilization, p. 616

64. 46, p. 616
65. Estrogen, p. 616
66. Progesterone, p. 616
67. Secondary sexual characteristics, p. 616
68. Menstrual cycle, p. 616
69. Puberty, p. 616

Choose the Correct Structure

70. A, p. 618
71. B, p. 618
72. C, p. 618
73. B, p. 618
74. A, p. 617
75. B, p. 617
76. A, p. 617
77. A, p. 617
78. C, p. 618

Matching
Group A

79. D, p. 618
80. E, p. 618
81. B, p. 619
82. C, p. 619
83. A, p. 619

Group B

84. E, p. 619
85. A, p. 619
86. D, p. 620
87. B, p. 620
88. C, p. 620

True or False

89. F (Menarche), p. 620
90. F (One), p. 622
91. F (14), p. 622
92. F (Menstrual period), p. 622
93. T
94. F (Anterior), p. 622

Choose the Correct Hormone

95. B, p. 622
96. A, p. 622
97. B, p. 622
98. B, p. 622
99. A, p. 622

Choose the Correct Response

100. F, p. 624
101. E, p. 624
102. A, p. 624
103. H, p. 624
104. I, p. 619

105. G, p. 624
106. C, p. 624
107. B, p. 622
108. L, p. 628
109. D, p. 623
110. J, p. 626
111. K, p. 628

Applying What You Know

112. Yes. The testes are not only essential organs of reproduction, but are also responsible for the "masculinizing" hormone. Without this hormone, Sam will have no desire to reproduce.
113. Sterile. The sperm count may be too low to reproduce but the remaining testicle will produce enough masculinizing hormone to prevent impotency.
114. The uterine tubes are not attached to the ovaries and infections can exit at this area and enter the abdominal cavity.
115. Yes. Without the hormones from the ovaries to initiate the menstrual cycle, Mrs. Harlan will no longer have a menstrual cycle and can be considered to be in menopause (cessation of menstrual cycle).
116. No. Vicki still will have her ovaries, which are the source of her hormones. She will not experience menopause due to this procedure.

117. **WORD FIND**

Crossword

```
¹A        ²C L I T O R I S
 M         I
 E      ³A R E O L A      ⁴P
 N         C              R
 O         U        ⁵S E M E N
 R      ⁶G A M E T E S    P
 R         C        ⁷V U L V A
 H        ⁸M       ⁹G     C
¹⁰T E S T O S T E R O N E
 A         I        N     N
           O        A     A
           N        D     D
           S        S     S
```

Male Reproductive Organs

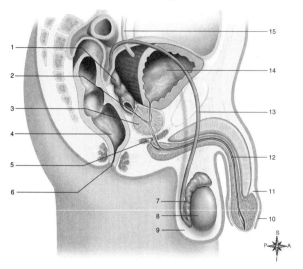

1. Seminal vesicle
2. Ejaculatory duct
3. Prostate gland
4. Rectum
5. Bulbourethral (Cowper) gland
6. Anus
7. Epididymis
8. Testis
9. Scrotum
10. Foreskin (prepuce)
11. Penis
12. Urethra
13. Ductus (vas) deferens
14. Urinary bladder
15. Ureter

Check Your Knowledge

Multiple Choice

1. A, p. 620
2. D, p. 622
3. D, p. 610
4. C, p. 612
5. C, p. 614
6. A, p. 605
7. B, p. 605
8. C, p. 611
9. A, p. 619
10. D, p. 627

Completion

11. C, p. 618
12. L, p. 605
13. H, p. 610
14. G, p. 617
15. F, p. 609
16. K, p. 611
17. B, p. 618
18. D, p. 616
19. J, p. 622
20. I, p. 622

Tubules of Testis and Epididymis

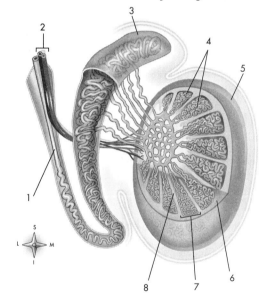

1. Ductus (vas) deferens
2. Nerves and blood vessels in the spermatic cord
3. Epididymis
4. Seminiferous tubules
5. Testis
6. Tunica albuginea
7. Lobule
8. Septum

Vulva

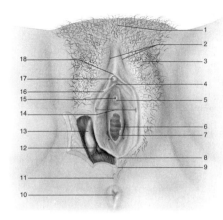

1. Mons pubis
2. Pudendal fissure
3. Labium majus
4. Frenulum (of clitoris)
5. Opening of lesser vestibular (Skene) gland
6. Orifice of vagina
7. Hymen
8. Frenulum (of labia)
9. Posterior commissure (of labia)
10. Anus
11. Perineum
12. Greater vestibular (Bartholin) gland
13. Vestibule (clitoral bulb)
14. Vestibule
15. External urinary meatus
16. Labium minus
17. Clitoris (glans)
18. Foreskin (prepuce)

Female Pelvis

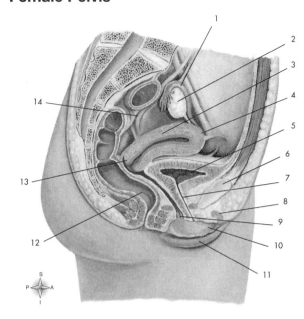

1. Uterine (fallopian) tube
2. Ovary
3. Body of uterus
4. Fundus of uterus
5. Urinary bladder
6. Symphysis pubis
7. Urethra
8. Clitoris
9. Vagina
10. Labium minus
11. Labium majus
12. Rectum
13. Cervix
14. Ureter

Breast

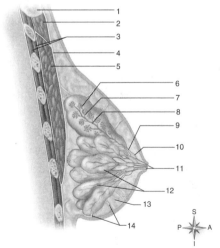

1. Clavicle
2. Pectoralis minor muscle
3. Intercostal muscle
4. Fascia of pectoral muscles
5. Pectoralis major muscle
6. Alveolus
7. Ductule
8. Duct
9. Lactiferous duct
10. Lactiferous sinus
11. Nipple pores
12. Lobes
13. Adipose tissue
14. Suspensory ligaments (of Cooper)

Uterus and Adjacent Structures

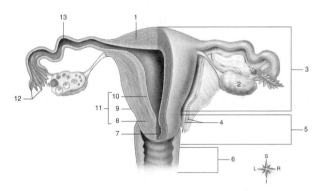

1. Fundus
2. Ovary
3. Body of uterus
4. Uterine artery and vein
5. Cervix
6. Vagina (cut)
7. Cervical canal
8. Myometrium
9. Perimetrium
10. Endometrium
11. Wall of uterus
12. Fimbriae
13. Uterine (fallopian) tube

CHAPTER 23
Growth and Development

Fill in the Blanks
1. Conception, p. 639
2. Birth, p. 639
3. Embryology, p. 640
4. Oviduct, fallopian tube, or uterine tube, p. 640
5. Zygote, p. 640
6. Morula, p. 640
7. Blastocyst, p. 641
8. Amniotic cavity, p. 642
9. Chorion, p. 642
10. Placenta, p. 642

Choose the Correct Term
11. G, p. 643
12. F, p. 644
13. C, p. 650
14. B, p. 643
15. A, p. 643
16. H, p. 647
17. E, p. 647
18. D, p. 645
19. I, p. 643
20. J, p. 650

True or False
21. T
22. T
23. F (Placenta previa), p. 649
24. F (Abruptio placentae), p. 649
25. F (Preeclampsia), p. 649
26. F (Stillbirth), p. 649
27. T

Multiple Choice
28. E, p. 651
29. E, p. 652
30. E, p. 653
31. A, p. 653
32. B, p. 653
33. C, p. 653
34. B, p. 653
35. D, p. 653
36. E, p. 653
37. D, p. 653
38. A, p. 653
39. C, p. 653
40. C, p. 653
41. C, p. 653
42. E, p. 653

Matching
43. F, p. 651

44. A, p. 652
45. C, p. 653
46. H, p. 653
47. D, p. 653
48. B, p. 652
49. E, p. 653
50. G, p. 654
51. I, p. 655

Fill in the Blanks
52. Lipping, p. 656
53. Osteoarthritis, p. 656
54. Nephron, p. 656
55. Barrel chest, p. 656
56. Atherosclerosis, p. 656
57. Arteriosclerosis, p. 656
58. Hypertension, p. 657
59. Presbyopia, p. 657
60. Cataract, p. 657
61. Glaucoma, p. 657

Unscramble the Words
62. Infancy
63. Postnatal
64. Organogenesis
65. Zygote
66. Childhood
67. Fertilization

Applying What You Know
68. Normal
69. Only about 40% of the taste buds present at age 30 remain at age 75.
70. A significant loss of hair cells in the organ of Corti causes a serious decline in ability to hear certain frequencies.
71. Each baby girl had her own placenta.

72. **WORD FIND**

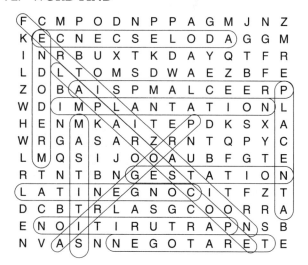

Crossword

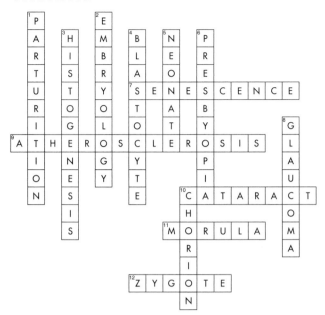

Fertilization and Implantation

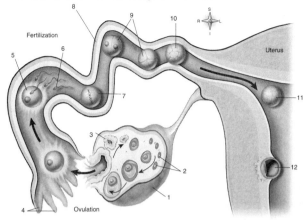

1. Ovary
2. Developing follicles
3. Corpus luteum
4. Fimbriae
5. Discharged ovum
6. Spermatozoa
7. First mitosis
8. Uterine (fallopian) tube
9. Divided zygote
10. Morula
11. Blastocyst
12. Implantation

Check Your Knowledge
Multiple Choice

1. C, p. 640
2. D, p. 656
3. D, p. 654
4. A, p. 652
5. D, p. 656
6. D, p. 657
7. A, p. 658
8. A, p. 654
9. C, p. 654
10. B, p. 644

Matching

11. E, p. 656
12. G, p. 656
13. C, p. 647
14. I, p. 657
15. H, p. 653
16. D, p. 642
17. J, p. 657
18. F, p. 655
19. A, p. 657
20. B, p. 642

CHAPTER 24
Genetics and Genetic Diseases

Matching
1. E, p. 666
2. A, p. 666
3. B, p. 668
4. C, p. 668
5. D, p. 668
6. G, p. 666
7. I, p. 666
8. J, p. 667
9. H, p. 667
10. F, p. 668

Fill in the Blanks
11. Genes, p. 669
12. Dominant, p. 669
13. Recessive, p. 669
14. Carrier, p. 669
15. Co-dominance, p. 670
16. Sex, p. 670
17. Female, p. 670
18. Mutation, p. 671
19. Genetic mutation, p. 671

Matching
20. E, p. 674
21. D, p. 672
22. J, p. 672
23. F, p. 674

24. C, p. 673
25. G, p. 675
26. A, p. 674
27. H, p. 675
28. B, p. 672
29. I, p. 676

Multiple Choice

30. D, p. 676
31. B, p. 677
32. C, p. 678
33. C, p. 677
34. D, p. 678
35. D, p. 680
36. B, p. 679

True or False

37. T
38. F (Electrophoresis), p. 679
39. F (Gene augmentation), p. 679
40. T
41. T

Unscramble the Words

42. Carrier
43. Trisomy
44. Gene
45. Pedigree
46. Chromosome
47. Inherited

Applying What You Know

48. In a form of dominance called *co-dominance*, the effect will be equal, causing "light brown" to occur.
49. One in four or 25%
50. Amniocentesis or chorionic villus sampling. The counselor will then produce a karyotype to determine anomalies.
51. **PUNNETT SQUARE**
    Mr. Fortner PP
    Mrs. Fortner pp
    a. 100% chance of brown eyes and 0% chance of blue eyes
    b. Yes
    c. 25%
    Mrs. Harrington Pp
    Mr. Harrington Pp
    a. Normal pigmentation 25%
    b. Carriers 50%
    c. Albinism 25%

52. **WORD FIND**

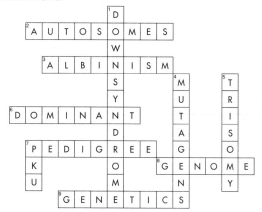

Crossword

Check Your Knowledge
Multiple Choice

1. A, p. 668
2. D, p. 676
3. C, p. 669
4. B, p. 668
5. A, p. 668
6. C, p. 666
7. B, p. 670
8. C, p. 670
9. A, p. 675
10. B, p. 676

Completion

11. H, p. 678
12. K, p. 678
13. C, p. 674
14. E, p. 666 (Review Chapter 3)
15. A, p. 674
16. G, p. 676
17. D, p. 669
18. J, p. 674
19. L, p. 674
20. B, p. 675